CHAKRA
FOR BEGINNERS

THE ULTIMATE GUIDE TO IMPROVE YOUR HEALTH,

HEAL YOURSELF AND BALANCE YOUR CHAKRAS

Table of Contents

INTRODUCTION

Almost all individuals in the western world are unfamiliar with what the Chakras are and how they impact our everyday lives, including our health. The captivating thing concerning Chakras is that, they play a big role in your emotional, spiritual and of course physical health. Chakras are simply energy facilities inside the body. This ancient Sanskrit word actually translates as "wheels of light".

These wheels of light are located vertically at the middle of your body, adapting around along with your backbone. Even when you're new to finding out more about alternative medicine and holistic health, or other spiritual thoughts and theosophical pursuits, using a solid comprehension of this complex energy system will definitely benefit everybody. Our bodies operate optimally when we have balanced and open Chakras.

When there's an imbalance or a blockage, the energy becomes trapped and can stagnate. This contributes to disease from the entire body, and when we don't re-establish the stream of energy, it may manifest as physical symptoms.

Chakras can be clarified as places in our body where the life-force(kundalini) is concentrated and contributes to tangible experiences on the emotional, physical and spiritual levels.

Everyone has life-force/ kundalini energy to a certain extent, so in everybody the Chakras are active to a degree and can be felt either at a gratifying manner or within a painful and distorted way. There are numerous systems and theories in various civilizations of the world concerning the various Chakras and energy channels in our body

Chakras have their vibrational frequency, own color, and symbol. For instance, the first Chakra is actually discovered at the base of the spinal column and it's described as the root Chakra. This particular Chakra governs the legs, kidneys, spinal column, rectum, feet, and immune system.

When the 1st Chakra is imbalanced, it leads to leg cramps, rectal problems, varicose veins, lower back pain, depression and immune related disorders. An out of balance root Chakra could be brought on by thoughts of self-esteem that is low, family concerns or insecurity. Some relevant Chakras are the heart, solar plexus, sacral, brow, throat, and crown Chakras.

Every energy center has to be vibrating at the right frequency independent of one another as a way for the whole body to vibrate in harmony. Thus, each Chakra is also crucial to optimum performance of the entire body based on the Chakra healing tradition. A lot of effective tools are able to influence the vibration of the Chakra, and that's where Chakra balancing is necessary.

Chakra stones, chants, music, human voice, mantras and meditation bring the Chakras frequency back to correct vibrational alignment. Chances are that you already possess a little awareness about the word 'Chakras'. Maybe you've seen or overheard conversations, pictures or gently dabbled in the energy systems of your body.

Based on practitioners of Chakra healing, all of us have 7 main Chakras which match with important aspects of the bodies and spiritual and emotional aspects of lives. The 7 Chakras form a line by the base of the backbone to the top part of the mind. Each Chakra represents a specific area of the human body.

As you learn how each affects your health, you could find out how to improve the quality of your overall state by opening, rebuilding, strengthening, and understanding your Chakras. Our objective is to have all those Chakras opened, balanced, and harmoniously working together.

These seven Chakras, along with hundreds of Chakras tend to draw of the coded information available from the environment. This coded info might be anything like color vibration beams, microwaves or another individual's aura. The 7 Chakras of the body are linked in different physical, emotional, psychological and spiritual levels.

The Chakras control a gland or organ on the level, and this controller is invisible with the frequency. This is because most of the glands, organs and body systems are attached to a Chakra that is linked to specific color vibration frequency.

These energy channels are not a mechanical system of pipes and vents within our own body by which energy flows but are highly individual experiences on the physiological, emotional and spiritual levels. In other words, everyone has slightly different experiences of their Chakras in their body.

The very first step required as a beginner is to understand that these 'wheels of light' also exist and then we must take the next step of learning how to open and balance our Chakras. Let's get started.

PART 1
INTRODUCING THE
CHAKRAS

CHAPTER 1

WHAT ARE CHAKRAS?

Chakras are simply energy facilities inside the body. This ancient Sanskrit word actually translates as "wheels of light".

These wheels of light are located vertically at the middle of your body, adapting around along with your backbone. The Chakras serve as energy transmitters from one level to another, distributing prana or qi into the physical body.

While there exist some minor Chakras in our joints and the body, it's understood that there exist seven major Chakras involving the top of the mind and the groin, with 2 others who are of major importance located about eighteen inches over the surface of the head, called the Earth Star and Soul Star, situated eighteen inches beneath the feet.

There are different views as to where few minor Chakras are. Our bodies operate optimally when our Chakras are balanced and open.

When there's an imbalance or a blockage, the energy becomes trapped and can stagnate. This contributes to disease from the entire body, and when we don't re-establish the stream of energy, it may manifest as physical symptoms.

Chakras can be clarified as places in our body where the life-force (kundalini) is concentrated and contributes to tangible experiences on the emotional, physical and spiritual levels.

Everyone has life-force/ kundalini energy to a certain extent, so in everybody the Chakras are active to a degree and can be felt either at a gratifying manner or within a painful and distorted way. There are numerous systems and theories in various civilizations of the world concerning the various Chakras and energy channels in the body.

The Hindu system acknowledges seven main Chakras, while the Tibetan Buddhist system speaks only of five. Yet, other systems explain three, nine or even twelve main Chakras. The ancient Indian mystics see the body centers as spinning, wheel-like vortices of energy. This chapter will provide you the Chakras synopsis and their role in the body.

When you fully understand exactly how every Chakra affects your physical functioning, you will be able to better decide which ones could be blocked or perhaps congested, and then work on balancing that Chakra. There are 7 major Chakras which are situated within the physical body in the base of our spine to the peak of the head, vertically aligned upwards and downwards the backbone.

They're tied into our nervous system along the backbone, various glands and endocrine system. The Chakras are also linked to different body functions such as breathing and digestion. In Tibetan Buddhism, the centers are known as station wheels. Taoist yoga is complex and dependent on the controller and the circulation of all vital energies found as vortexes.

Chakras, also referred to as lotuses, give us a notion of Chakra nature. The lotus and its beautiful flowers blooming on the water surface, beneath the sunlight (spirit) buries its roots in the muddy shadow of the depths (physical). As the lotus blossoms, Chakras can be opening, closing or blossoming, in bud, dormant or active.

The old alchemical tradition used the new system, with planets as well as metals being given to the Chakras inside an intricate system, which formed the foundation of the pursuit for spiritual transformation.

With all the drop of alchemical arts, understanding of the Chakras disappeared also. Fascination with the Chakras reemerged in the west together with the look of the theosophy action in the late nineteenth as well as early twentieth centuries.

The Chakra process is an energetic information storage method, very similar to a computer, system that many folks see or feel. It is the religious interface existing between our physical body, our spirit body, and the nervous system. The nervous system, of course, is our physical interface, relaying information with all areas of the physical, providing information to receiving out of the Chakras.

Personal experience is a crucial part of the western endorsement for all, our "I will only believe it if I see it" syndrome, and likewise constraints to our multi-sensory experiences. There are many incidences however, where individuals have experienced body pain at the center, without a real reason discovered, even after thorough medical testing.

When these people went on to have a Chakra balance and crystal recovery, the healer found their pain to be linked to a past life accident and also the pain resolved after the balancing. Many healers think that physical disorders have their root in psychological and mental imbalances. So, to heal the physical body, you must also cover the emotional and psychological area as well.

Each of the popularly known seven Chakras directly corresponds to the physical system and its associated glands and organs. Colors, sounds and crystals are designated to each Chakra, though the functions and color of each Chakra varies based on different traditions.

CHAPTER 2
HISTORY OF CHAKRA

Most people believe that the 7 Chakras comes from the Hindu and Buddhist customs. Even though it's correct that they were written about from the Upanishads, an ancient Vedic text from India which was written in Sanskrit between 1500 and 500 B.C., understanding of the Chakras is thought to be more historical than the Vedic texts. Egyptians had been practicing them until they were passed to the Yogis and Buddhists of Southeast Asia.

The Ethiopians thought that understanding of the Chakras was passed from Tanzania. From that point, the ancient Egyptians are the first to benefit from the healing and spiritual comprehension of the 7 Chakras.

Afterwards, this understanding was released to India as individuals traveled west, where it flourished and has been listed in the Sanskrit texts known as the Upanishads. Most from the western world are unfamiliar with what Chakras are, and how they impact our everyday lives, such as our wellness.

The attractive thing about Chakras is that they play a major part in your emotional, religious and of course wellness. The ancient Indians find out strange spirals of light thousands of years ago. This light, also known as CHAKRAS, is a topic of interest to many individuals nowadays in search of deeper knowledge.

These Chakras are considered a means of ridding the body of negative energy forces and renewing the energy of an individual. A Chakra relates to and broadcasts the power of life force; it is the effort of position within the body. Charka comes from the Sanskrit word which describes a continuously spinning wheel or the sphere aural power we each have.

Lots of standard Hindu writings suggest that there are close to a hundred thousand points of Chakra all through an individual's body. Although, you will find 7 Chakras that happen to be much more critical than many of the others. These Chakras are available to the lower part of the backbone all the way up to the roof of the mind.

These 7 major Chakras receive and transmit signals to and from the common surroundings or the infinite Cosmos. They influence the religious, intellectual, emotional, mystical, psychological and corporeal state of a person. Chakras have been discussed in different methods, but most of those descriptions have one common characteristic.

May it be through the Chinese medicinal point of view or the Hindu point of view these explanations are, in fact, all similar. It is the understanding of the experiences of individuals and the way that the human brain believes and goes through numerous emotions. The Hindu system acknowledges seven main Chakras, while the Tibetan Buddhist system speaks only of five.

Yet, other systems explain three, nine or even twelve main Chakras. These seven Chakras, along with hundreds of Chakras tend to draw of the coded information available from the environment. This coded info could be anything like color vibration beams, microwaves or another individual's aura.

The 7 Chakras of the body are linked to the body in different physical, emotional, psychological and spiritual levels. The Chakras control a gland or organ on the level, and this controller is invisible with the frequency. This is because most of glands, organs and body systems are attached to a Chakra which are likewise connected to the specific color vibration frequency.

All seven Chakras are aligned on the column; and every disturbance to any one of these Chakras reflects an alteration at their level. Moreover, each has its own intelligence center that controls the body's psychological, physiological and belief system. Each Chakra can also be balanced by using a Chakra (color) vibration of the exact same frequency.

Chakras that are imbalanced indicate that the Chakras are under or overactive or they are congested or blocked. This imbalance is sensed on a physical, psychological or emotional level and is credited to pollutants like poor environmental factors, negative ideas and the compound. As this imbalance can't be treated by health care procedures, we must comprehend our Chakra system to boost our health requirements.

The significance of understanding our Chakra system is what makes it possible to understand Chakras as a whole. This whole means the harmonic relation between mind, spirit and body. Some believe that understanding Chakras is the key to achieving wonderful states of serene, lively bliss.

The secret that eludes so many is the way to find and release these forces that lie somewhere deep within the self. Chakra is an ancient concept that originally appeared in the Sanskrit (Indian holy writing). Now it's used to explain a belief in wellness and health that science fails to completely clarify.

There are many writings about Chakra and the concept transgresses throughout health, energy and religion. However, we will concentrate more on its relation. Chakra is the energy that connects mind, human body and soul into a single. Many writings about this mysterious belief indicates that Chakra is at the middle of convergence for lifetime energy for humans.

There are six (or seven in other writings and beliefs) Chakra points on the body and each stage corresponds to a point where we assimilate, manifest and receive energy. Chakra centers are situated on different locations of the spine. It branches through our body starting from the base of the column and up towards the top of our skull.

Even If we're to discover new learnings about holistic health and alternative medicine or other spiritual thoughts and pursuits that are theosophical, everybody will be surely benefiting by utilizing an in-depth knowledge of the energy system.

Chakras are utilized in therapeutic applications and in meditation. Their energy is directly believed to have the capacity to rid the body of energies associated with sadness and disease.

There are lots of other advantages to be found beyond these applications while some people become interested in this force for a way to relieve their worldly aches, pains and sorrows. After the Chakras are understood by you as a whole, they start communicating and working in cooperation with one another to leave energy issues to you.

So, once the part of your body is powerful, your psychological, physical and spiritual elements are also strong to leave you feeling at the best. The issue is that life renders many people with no time to comprehend these Chakras as a whole. People are inclined to emphasize more on Chakras, which are exactly what leads to many health, mental and emotional problems in people.

CHAPTER 3
THE SCIENCE BEHIND CHAKRAS

There are hundreds of minor Chakras or energy points across the human body. All these minor and major Chakras draw in info from the frequency vibrations out of our surroundings. This information can be another person's air, astral radiation or simply anything that gives a vibrational frequency, which can be everything based on modern physics.

The point is, our Chakras let us comprehend how healthy our surroundings are. This includes the folks as well as animals we come in contact with. The Chakras of ours may even produce a vibrational energy of their own. Of the 7 major Chakras we have, each is connected to us spiritually, psychologically, mentally and physically.

The bodily link of this Chakra regulates a various gland or organ which, in turn, regulates another body part or function of the human body. There's not an organ, gland or system within the body that isn't connected to some Chakra.

In turn each Chakra is consequently placed on a vibrational color frequency. In order to provide you with a good example, the heart Chakra vibrational frequency is going green.

This Chakra regulates the bronchia system, heart, lungs, lymph glands, immune system, with the arms as well as hands. These primary Chakras are arranged alongside the spinal column.

The Chakras energy level will demonstrate any disturbances that may happen in the body, mind or soul. In addition, each of the 7 major Chakras functions as its own intellect processing center.

This has wide range consequences as it means that Chakra isn't only connected to certain organs or glands, but it will also control aspects of our mental and psychological health. The best part is we can balance or tune the Chakras of ours. This may be done by introducing the Chakra vibrational color that is at exactly the identical frequency as the Chakra we wish to balance.

This can be done in order to help improve our spiritual, emotional, mental, and physical state. The human air will resonate the various colors of the Chakras. If we understand what these colors mean we've got the needed information to correctly balance our Chakras. If a Chakra is imbalanced, it may affect other surrounding Chakras along with the different parts of the human body they regulate.

An out of balance Chakra indicates that it's overactive or underactive. The Chakra congested or could be blocked somehow. When your Chakras are imbalanced it is also possible to feel it on all levels of your body assuming you are in contact with your body. Whether we are awake or not, the Chakras are actually in continuous motion.

This particular continuous exercise is going to influence the framework, looks, body disorders, glandular procedures in addition to our deeds and thoughts. Nevertheless, if there's a Chakra malfunction in a single or more points, which could be brought on by different reasons, an imbalance will develop that will help make itself acknowledged in other parts of our being. It is thought that this is because of the Chakras being attached to the endocrine system in the body.

So long as a Chakra gets off balance at all, we can experience what is known as a disturbance in the standard actions of the endocrine gland and all that's connected to it.

You can easily say some serious ailments or illnesses that the body might be suffering may be connected to an unbalanced Chakra. It is necessary to keep the correct Chakra stability so you can keep your body working properly.

While you might not see some actual physical characteristics of an imbalance or an illness, you might see a positive change in the emotions. One of the primary factors behind Chakra imbalance is the repressed or forgotten mental baggage we carry because of those previous traumatic experiences.

Many people habitually bury the awful memories into the subconscious mind of theirs, unaware that these psychological harmful toxins which are buried within them are going to influence the bodies in a cellular state

Thus, it is crucial to cope with emotional baggage once and for those who can keep a good balancing of the Chakras which ignites a healing process to start on the actual physical person. You have to recognize that Chakra healing is great for the human body so you can directly impact every single one of the Chakras.

You can employ methods like aromatherapy, Reiki healing, Chakra balancing, color therapy, with the aid of a pendulum, gemstones or crystals. When you have painful or stressful experiences from the past (even the latest past) which never got healed, they are hanging around in the energy field like they are never going on and could hinder the good thoughts and experiences you wish to have in the present. Ultimately, additionally, they interfere with wellness.

There are 7 major Chakras which are located to the peak of the mind, vertically aligned upwards and downwards the backbone within the physical body at the spine base.

They are directly tied to the nervous system with the backbone, various glands and endocrine system. The Chakras can also be linked to various bodily functions such as digestion and breathing. Chakras are also called lotuses and that gives us an idea of Chakra nature.

The lotus with its exquisite blossoms blooming on the water surface, under the sun (soul) buries its origins in the muddy shadow of the depths (physical). As the blossom can be shut, starting or blossoming, in active, dormant or bud.

The early alchemical tradition utilizes the system, with planets and metals that are assigned to each Chakra in an elaborate system, which formed the cornerstone of the quest for transformation spiritually. The Chakra system is also known as energy storage system, very similar to a computer that many people feel or see.

It is the religious interface between our soul body and the physical body, along with also the nervous system. The system naturally is our physical interface, communication with all areas of the physical, providing information to getting out of the 7 Chakras. The Chakras serve as energy transmitters from one level to another, distributing prana or qi to our physical body.

While there are many other Chakras within our joints and the body, it is known there are 7 basic Chakras between the surface of the mind and the groin with two others that are of big importance located about eighteen inches over the surface of the mind, called the Earth Star, and Soul Star, situated approximately 18 inches beneath the toes. There are various views as to where few of the Chakras are.

Experience is a crucial part of western endorsement for all, our, "I can only believe it If I see it" syndrome, and also limits to our multi-sensory experiences. There are many incidences where folks have experienced body pain, at the heart with no real reason found, even after comprehensive medical testing.

When these folks went to have a Chakra balance and crystal recovery, the healer discovered their pain to be linked to a past life accident and the pain resolved after the balancing. Many healers believe that physical disorders get their root in psychological and psychological imbalances.

Thus, for you to cure the physical body, you must also cover the emotional and psychological area too. Each of the commonly known seven Chakras corresponds to the physical system and its associated glands and organs. Colors, crystals and sounds are designated to each Chakra, though the functions and color of each Chakra fluctuates based on various traditions.

The seven major Chakras represent the 4 elements -- fire, earth, air and water and sound, thought and light. Each Chakra is indicated by a single color of the seven colors of the rainbow -- red, indigo, orange, yellow, blue, green, and purple. These centers are also correlated with the various glands and organs within the human body. Each of the Chakras has a different task when it comes to physical operation.

Additionally, your personality is affected by each Chakra too. When these Chakras are balanced and clear, equally your emotional, physical and spiritual bodies might benefit. Chakra clearing may be a superb tool for obtaining a sense of well-being and improved health.

Every Chakra is related to a certain color and physical and emotional connection. For instance, lower Chakras are actually linked with back pain. They also envelope physic energies that are utilized for materializations and mediums for creating ectoplasm. Just like the heart Chakra is among the 7 Chakras. The designated color is going green. It is related to the emotions encompassing love.

As the middle of the main Chakras, it links the lower Chakras with the top ones. Generally, a well-nourished heart Chakra results to love that is unconditional for yourself and some close to you.

It can additionally be spiritual or divine love. The imbalanced heart Chakra can cause an individual to be delicate leading him to feel negative feelings for example heart troubles, depression, coldness, and anger.

Individuals with imbalanced heart Chakras have difficulties associated with romantic relationships. This is since they might provide but expect nothing in exchange.

CHAPTER 4

THE BENEFITS OF DIFFERENT CHAKRAS

Each Chakra is also relatively associated with various body parts, colors, emotions, along with other features. Let's look at the benefits of the 7 Chakras in turn, beginning from the first to the seventh in comprehensive details.

Root Chakra

The very first of the 7 Chakras of the body is referred to as the root Chakra. Chakra is a Sanskrit term which signifies wheel, in addition to the Sanskrit name of the very first Chakra is 'mujadara' which suggests root or base. This particular Chakra, as the title indicates, is found in the foundation in between the genitals as well as anus.

Because there's energy stored within this Chakra, it is frequently called the serpent. It is likely by focusing on it through Kundalini yoga, to excite and renew this energy as this is the first Chakra where energy is obtained from the seven individual Chakras. This is actually the center of bodily energy and is regarded as the energy foundation of the body.

As soon as you understand how you can connect with the chart, you discover that it's simple as it guides you on the journey of your life to nourish your spiritual and physical needs.

It is important that this Chakra function is to assist the free flow of energy to and out of the human body. When in equilibrium, life is thought by you to maintain equilibrium and can be working stably.

A root Chakra possesses a security feeling and keeps filling you with energy that is active. It is this energy which produces a solid sense to keep and preserve good relationships. Sometimes, the Chakra may be out of balance. You begin feeling a reduction in your sense of belonging if the Chakra is at equilibrium.

Some people even start feeling more worried about their own survival and safety when their first Chakra is imbalanced. The harshness of these feelings in people is dependent upon what they had previously gone through in their own lives. Some people can also experience melancholy, suffer from deficiency of self-esteem, get confused in addition to kidney issues, pain in legs and feet and disconnection.

With meditation and yoga which target the 1st Chakra, it is very likely to boost your wellness and to start the blockages up at the 1st Chakra. You will begin to feel grounded and focused and start to experience prosperity. It's related to this basic potentiality, safety and survival.

Hence, it's acceptable to contact this Chakra to the Root or maybe Muladhara Service. The significance of the Chakra is that it governs equilibrium - Mental, Emotional, Physical and also other kinds of equilibrium. That is where you get the expression "You have to get a backbone!" from. It is often known as the cycle is repeated in addition to the previous point of those nadi.

As soon as you started feeling a sense of life, rest, organized and practical, you will find it a whole lot easier to take care of harm and any trouble that might come your way.

The Sacral Chakra implies the 'living area of self'.

The sacral Chakra is located at the lower belly, about an inch below the navel. The organs connected to the sacral Chakra are the kidneys, low back, hips, sacrum and all body fluids like urine, blood, tears and childbirth.

As this Chakra is profoundly associated with procreation, imagination and controls all matters in life, all your sexual energy lies here. That's the sole reason why those who have a second Chakra knowingly or unknowingly sensually attract others, such as the film stars that are numerous. The Sacral Chakra can also lead to some sexual addiction. In reality, a Sacral Chakra has overactive adaptation to sex.

Everything they do and believe, revolves around intercourse, like a sexual addiction. The Chakra can get overactive when they reside in an environment with continuous requirement for satisfying stimulation such as constant caring and enjoyment and also an environment of routine or psychological drama. A balanced Sacral Chakra manifests when the person lives a life that is healthy to enhance their sexual energy.

But in circumstances in which the person grew up in an environment where their feelings are refused or suppressed, they begin dreading for pleasure, get rid of contact with their feelings and withstand shifting.

A well balanced second Chakra generates a capacity for creativity and partnerships with individuals. Your brain gets devoid of any anxieties. However, once the Chakra is imbalanced, you begin developing psychological problems connected with sex.

You begin to develop guilt feelings and start finding it hard to get without really getting jumped. You typically give others from responsibility, instead of in the heart. You're likely to have to sleep a lot, only to find that you don't feel rested when you are awake as you're always at a chronic lack of energy.

To balance an imbalanced 2nd Chakra, you need to focus, eat and use orange-colored items, do especially yoga stances, eat a lot of candies and drink as much water as possible.

Solar Plexus

The third major Chakra of the entire body is generally known as the Manipura. It is a Sanskrit word that means 'gem'. This Chakra is located in the solar navel plexus and the digestive system area which is also the site of intelligence.

The solar plexus is related to self-esteem, energy, self-control, power and subject. People that have a solid 3rd Chakra tend to display characteristics such as a function in life, livelihood, internal power and self-confidence. The organs and glands connected to the solar plexus are the gastrointestinal tract and the pancreas.

That is the reason one starts growing digestive issues with imbalances in the solar plexus Chakra. The health problems that arise from an obstructed third Chakra are nausea, diabetes, hypoglycemia, digestive issues, over-sexuality, depression, muscular cramps, eating disorders, skin ailments and problems in the spleen, kidneys, pancreas and nerve cells.

With numerous health problems arising out of a third Chakra that is obstructed, experts say that the health complications could result in individuals getting obsessed with power. But when this Manipura Chakra is in equilibrium, the individual gains self-esteem spontaneity and develops a self-identity.

They produce a power that originates in the middle of their human body from the solar plexus area which makes them feel as if they belonged everywhere. It contributes to the functioning of assimilation, metabolism and food digestion. As people with a third strong Chakra are successful in their toes, specialists do agree that a variety of the greatest dancers have a potent third Chakra.

Heart Chakra

The 4th Chakra is situated in the middle of the torso behind the breastbone. This is the arena of connection, empathy, retrieval, compassion, affinity for others and self. The element connected to the Chakra is atmosphere.

Throughout our productive adulthood years, it should be regarded as pink, the integration of this white (function) color of the crown and the red (fire) color of the first melody. Ultimately, we would like to attain the love, gold color. This is the middle of affinity for others and yourself.

This is a result of advices we grew with; it's far better to give than receive, and we have to care for everyone else first and caring for ourselves is "egotistical". The reality of is that if we don't love and care for ourselves, we do not have love to give to anybody else. We live in the interior. The love we give ourselves fixes the norm for a healthy relationship, one where we get up to, we supply.

Everybody in this world is here to experience development, roughing their elbows up, falling down so that they could get up. That is exactly what we came for. What we could call mistakes are lessons to move forward and it is no one's obligation to protect someone else.

Parents might have a tricky time with this. The heart Chakra is responsible for our fantasies and desires. At the middle down the arms and out of the hands as healing energy flows, renewable energy does.

I have seen debilitating energy when creativity has been squelched.

Throat Chakra

This Chakra is the mean of communication and is closely connected to the soul into the reflection of its own needs. In my experience, the fifth Chakra goes deeper than simple communication.

Throughout the Chakra, we say who we are, what we are here for and what we desire and speak our truth. The purpose of the 5th Chakra is "the capability to define ourselves out of the entire world". This isn't necessarily easy to accomplish since the energy that's behind this saying is certainty and certainty comes from a sense of worth and value.

Unworthiness and invalidation are all energies that obstruct the Chakra. Perhaps in this life or past, it wasn't feasible to speak the truth out of fear of persecution, punishment or even death. This energy might be irrational in this present lifetime but the fears it arouses are extremely genuine and shut down that communicating center.

Another energy which blocks the 5th Chakra is responsible for estimating, censoring or swallowing the phrases in order to be approved by the person that we're speaking to if that is eventually great for us or not. I am not speaking about being socially okay I am speaking about not being loyal to yourself in order to eventually become "okay" with someone else or a group of individuals.

The 5th Chakra is the engine for discharging and processing emotion. "Discussing it" is a great explanation of talking through your emotions, which releases them in the physical body. The Yang or incoming purpose of the 5th Chakra is about expressing. Yin purpose or the open minded of the 5th Chakra is responsible for getting information.

Brow Center Chakra

The 6th Chakra is the inner control center. We can utilize this Chakra to understand what by making use of our imagination, we would like to encounter. This Chakra is also the location where we can detect what is happening in our lives with neutrality.

If you put consciousness or your attention into the sixth Chakra, you'll observe that you are just not at the emotion of the Chakra and may discover what is happening. You might be the observer.

With neutrality, you can view and act clearly. Within practice, we made a room within our six Chakras known as our "Center of Head Room". It's the place where we navigate clairvoyantly.

If you're not interested in clairvoyance, the center stage of the mind is a stunning place to make an inner sanctuary for prayer and meditation. The subject of moving into your inner sanctuary in order to communicate is valuable in my opinion.

Make it a place to be, inviting yourself personally and you will be fed and nurtured once you're there. Spirit speaks through creativity and drama, so the Chakra is a place where you can discover your soul through images. Energy that blocks the 6th Chakra is your view that imagination is counterproductive to achievement and may be a waste of time.

The Crown Center Chakra

It may be described as "the psychics hub" for increased comprehension, it receives the spiritual energies and advice required to trigger our goal. It includes the capability to live our celestial identity by expressing intention, along with the Yin capacity to take part in energies critical to feeding our religious character. As beings, Chakras include information from this lifetime in addition.

It is thought that the crown Chakra holds the information within the other Chakras. There are few kinds of energy which I see impeding the Chakra; one has to do with beliefs and principles and the other one with value. The spiritual kind of energy can receive data that we, as individuals, aren't able to assimilate advices. A variety of energies could be quite stern.

Another energy handling value has to do with understanding that we are celestial beings and advices and inspiration we are offered is our birthright. Information is coming continuously but unless we're accepting and are aware of it we won't receive it. How many times do we get a reply, request for help and question it or talk ourselves out of it entirely? We do not think we can have it.

The simple reality is that all of us are psychic although answers come to folks who are spiritual or believed by us to be psychic. The expression "psychic" is a Greek word and it just means "of the Spirit".

PART 2
VISUALIZATION OF YOUR CHAKRAS

CHAPTER 5
ROOT CHAKRA

The very first of the 7 Chakras of the human body is called the Root Chakra. Chakra is a Sanskrit word that translates as wheel, and the Sanskrit title of this primary Chakra is 'Muladhara' which signifies root or foundation. This Chakra is situated at the bottom of the backbone, between the anus and genitals. Because there is energy saved beneath this Chakra, the Chakra is frequently known as the coiled serpent.

It's likely to renew and excite this energy by focusing on it via Kundalini yoga. As this is the first of the 7 human Chakras, this is really where other Chakras obtain their power from. This is the middle of bodily energy and is regarded as the body's energy base.

As soon as you learn to connect to the chart, you find it simple to feed your physical and spiritual needs since it guides you on your life's journey. The Root Chakra is located at the lower part of the spine and is linked with the Saturn planet. Saturn represents our ability to emphasize our fantasies. Absence of Saturn in our lives hinders us to support ourselves.

For some, with little Saturn it is hard to create a sense of bounds, while with full Saturn, nevertheless, we could resist change due to insecurity and fear. One of the techniques of curing the 1st Chakra is via linking with the earth energies. Walking barefoot and practicing yoga are different ways of tuning at the first Chakra's lower frequencies.

Drumming is an effective method of stirring and launching the first Chakra. When the drum is held between our thighs, which instantly connects with the first Chakra at the spine base, we never energize ourselves but become bodies by tuning at the lower frequencies of the drum. Because there's energy stored within this Chakra, it is frequently called the serpent.

It is likely by focusing on it through Kundalini yoga, to excite and renew this energy as this is the 1st of the Chakras where energy is obtained from, for the seven individual Chakras. This is actually the center of bodily energy and is regarded as the energy foundation of the body. As soon as you understand the way to connect with the chart, you discover that it's simple as it guides you on the journey of your life to nourish your spiritual and physical needs. It is important that this Chakra function is to assist the free flow of energy to and out of the human body.

When in equilibrium, life can be working stably. The root Chakra offers a safety feeling and keeps filling you with energy that is active. It is this energy which produces a solid way of keeping and preserving good relationships. Sometimes, the Chakra may be out of balance.

You begin feeling a reduction in your sense of belonging if the Chakra is at equilibrium. Some people even start feeling more worried about their own survival and safety when their first Chakra is imbalanced. The harshness of these feelings in people is dependent upon what they have previously gone through in their lives.

Chakra color - RED

Utilizing red things such as clothes, red food and drinks helps awaken this Chakra. Visualizing red items such as a vibrant, deep red roses or a crimson hibiscus might awaken a soothing feeling inside you. Eating veggies and red fruits while still working on this Chakra helps greatly.

An obstructed root Chakra may make you feel like there is absolutely no help for your life. You experience low back pain. In addition, the symptom you encounter can be followed by blockages like polyps, varicose veins or tumors in the rectal region. Some people also suffer melancholy, suffer from deficiency of self-esteem, get confused in addition to kidney issues, pain in legs and feet or disconnection.

With meditation and yoga that target the 1st Chakra, it is very likely to boost your wellness and to start the blockages up at the 1st Chakra. You will begin to feel grounded and focused and start to experience prosperity. It's related to this basic potentiality, safety and survival. As most of us know, any damage to the spinal cord can result in irreversible damage our nervous system.

Thus, it right to name this Chakra the Root or Muladhara Service. The necessity of the Chakra resides in governing equilibrium - Mental, Emotional, Physical and also other kinds of equilibrium. That is where we get the expression "You have to get a backbone!". It is often known as the cycle is repeated in addition to the previous point of those nadi.

As soon as you started feeling a sense of life, rest, you will find it a whole lot easier to take care of harm and any upsets that may come your way. Essential Oils: Cinnamon, Peppermint, Cloves, Patchouli, Sandalwood.

Root Chakra is your 1st or base Chakra. It connects the soul and body and, in addition, our own body to mother earth. It's situated at the base of the spine.

This Chakra controls our instincts of self-preservation or survival. Particular areas of our personalities are attributed to the primordial Chakra such as the feelings of security and protection in addition to primal sexual urges.

When a root Chakra is balanced, we feel relaxed, wholesome and full of life, capable to accomplish tasks, lively, energetic, we believe that life is abundant, happy and we are sexually healthy. Due to unexpected circumstances such as the demise of a beloved one, the main Chakra could possibly be thrown off at times.

Events have a way of turning our world inside out and it's not surprising that our Chakras will be thrown off balance along with everything else. When the root Chakra is imbalanced, an individual may feel disconnected from oneself, afraid, victimized or prone to violent outbursts. It's important for this Chakra to be balanced, so it can assist the free flow of energy, to and out of the ground.

When in balance, you think life can also be in equilibrium and can be functioning stably. A balanced root Chakra gives a safety feeling and fills you with busy, optimistic energy. It's this positive energy that produces a strong power to keep and maintain good relationships with everybody. Sometimes, the first Chakra may head out of equilibrium.

When the 1st Chakra is at balance, you begin feeling disconnected from the others and reduce your sense of belonging. Some people even begin feeling more concerned with their own survival and security when their very first Chakra is imbalanced. The harshness of these feelings in people is dependent upon what they'd previously gone through in their lives.

Security and Safety

The Base or Root Chakra is physically situated at the perineum, the region between the vagina or testicles and the anus. Each Chakra resonate at different colors and notes. The Base Chakra's resonance when healthy can be viewed by the psychics as resonating to red and the psychic sound is actually the note C.

The base Chakra is centered on problems surrounding the subject matter of security and safety. Areas as cash, house, food, clothes, family, heritage, ancestry, one's place on Earth are both applicable to the Base Chakra. You will know if you are genuinely in balance with this Chakra if your security and safety are healthful without you having to think it over.

You are healthy. You don't feel unsafe or safe, you simply are healthy. You don't feel prosperous or concerned about money, you just usually have the necessary wealth to live life your way. You are never focused on cash especially, you simply like living life. In reality, the majority of us aren't actually that balanced regarding the base Chakra. The Western Society is especially out of stability in the areas of security and cash. You will find ways to bring the system back into balance, however. Here's a list: change the thinking - read books and watch movies based on the law of prosperity, consciousness and attraction. Training physical activities that give a spiritual connection to the body like Yoga, walking meditations and Chakra dance.

Spend some time in nature, even in the garden or the nearby park with the shoes off. Meditate with the aim of connecting to the Base Chakra. Question it way it feels and just what must be whole and healthy.

Put on red socks or even pants/underpants. Do frequent power work like Reiki self-treatments. Delve into the Chakra to fix or restore damage and trauma, fragmented soul parts with Advanced Energy Surgery (The Consciousness Call mentoring work). Visit the

Consciousness Call to discover the countless programs that could support the empowerment.

Building a relationship with the Base Chakra consists of building the consciousness around your relationship with money, safety, overall health and house. Begin with the experience around these various facets of life, look at life and search for possiblies, damaging encounters to see whether they have healed or even if there's work to be completed.

The greater you get to know the Base Chakra and also the elements of living it pertains to, the greater you can heal and empower and enhance the Self.

CHAPTER 6
SACRAL CHAKRA

The second Chakra is responsible for how we channel our basic life, force, energy and feelings and problems of creativity and novelty.

Jupiter is the planet that reflects our consciousness extent. If we grew in a family that suppressed feelings of sexuality, this could have immediately influenced the sense of expansiveness. Whenever this Chakra is open, we're linked with all our kundalini energy or life force that was primal.

This is the basic force that brings accurate creativity in our lives, fire, and magnetism that animates our bodies. The key to awakening the power of this Chakra is to extend the selection of motion and to acquire our energy moving and open. Any motions that contract and enlarge the area of the Chakra, will help release the energy.

Furthermore, using ethnic or world music to activate the instinctual or transferring center, such as didgeridoo, belly dancing or Turkish dervish songs are exceptional. This Chakra implies the 'living area of self'.

The sacral Chakra is located at the lower belly, about an inch below the navel. The organs and areas connected to the sacral Chakra are the kidneys, lower back, hips, sacrum and all body fluids like urine, blood, tears and childbirth.

As this Chakra is profoundly associated with procreation, imagination and controls all matters in life, all your sexual energy lies here. It's the reason why those that have a second Chakra knowingly or unknowingly sensually attract others. The Sacral Chakra can also lead to some sexual addiction.

Everything the individuals characterized by a strong second Chakra do and believe, revolve around intercourse, like a sexual addiction. The Chakra can get overactive when they reside in an environment with continuous requirement for satisfying stimulation or an environment of routine and psychological drama.

But in cases when the person grew up in an environment where their feelings were refused or suppressed, they begin dreading for pleasure, get rid of contact with their feelings and withstand shifting.

Color - Orange

Orange is the color for the second Chakra, which is an extremely arousing color because of its vibration energy.

Concentrating on orange items helps excite and clear any blockages you will experience in the 2nd Chakra. You should use a whole lot of orange to wake up the Chakra and consume more fruits like orange, peppers, mango and cantaloupe. This chart's element is Water which explains the reason you want to use water in every recovery you might consider.

You need to drink as much water as you please, the same as herbal teas as hibiscus blossom or chamomile. Some crystals that help balance the Chakra are garnet, carnelian, tiger's eye, amber, citrine, moonstone, rose quartz, orange zincite, fire agate, fire pit, topaz and coral. The feeling that arouses the Chakra is the sensation of flavor.

Thus, the foods you need to consume to stimulate the Chakra are orange foods that are sweet and contain lots of liquids. A balanced sacral Chakra generates a capacity for creativity and partnerships with individuals. Your brain gets devoid of any anxieties. However, once the Chakra is imbalanced, you begin developing psychological problems connected with sex.

What you give to others typically comes from a sense of responsibility, instead of coming from your heart. You're likely to have to sleep a lot, only to find that you don't feel rested as you're always at a chronic lack of energy.

To balance an imbalanced 2nd Chakra, you need to focus, eat and use orange-colored items, do special yoga stances, eat candies and drink as much water as possible. The sacral Chakra relates to sexuality and reproduction.

If this Chakra is imbalanced, your physical health may be at risk. The sacral Chakra is directly connected to the main Chakra. It's found a few fingers beneath the naval.

It's joined on the lymphatic system as well as adrenal glands. When the body is stressed, the adrenaline is released to keep it in a state of alert. It is essential to work with this Chakra when stressed. Balancing this Chakra is a requirement to help calming the central nervous system.

Emotionally, this Chakra corresponds to our feelings of well-being. This Chakra likewise promotes clairsentience which is a psychic ability. It enables a psychic reader to hold an item or touch somebody and sense the energy surrounding that place, person or thing.

Essential Oils: Patchouli, Rose, Sage, Bergamot, Ylang-Ylang, Sandalwood

The Sacral Chakra is located just below the belly button in the lower abdominal area. It governs heritage and emotions. A balanced sacral Chakra assures a wonderful sexual energy as well as a great awareness for our own emotions.

If the sacral Chakra is imbalanced, you might constantly feel either too emotional or needy or, on the opposite end of the spectrum, totally disconnected from people and emotionally down.

Many other signs of an imbalance include fear of intimacy, infidelity and sexual dysfunction. The sacral Chakra regulates creativity and our power. You need to press at just two inches down your navel.

A blockage may lead to resistance to unique ideas. An open sacral Chakra is very evident and in all reckless behavior, ranges from dangerous driving to bed-hopping.

Sacral Chakra Crystal Correction: Carnelian, a beautiful quarz.

The stimulating qualities of orange or red gives courage to the timid even though it can be discovered in several colors. This allow us to pursue our great dreams, excluding fear-based illusions obstructing our path.

Conversely, if this really is too open, you may require "luizi". This blue stone was valued in Babylon and ancient Egypt. We can utilize its properties to help us act with caution these days.

Only touching your system with this rock improves your spiritual, psychic, mental, physical, and psychological condition. For optimal benefits to the sacral Chakra, you need to allow this stone to rest.

A developed sacral Chakra guarantees the wellness of the reproductive system, prostate, testicles, uterus and ovaries, urinary tract, pelvis, small intestine, lower vertebrae, cecum, ileum, duodenum, bladder. Additionally, it stops impotence and lowers menstrual ache.

A powerful sacral Chakra can help in the assimilation of meals, strengthen the immune system and detoxify the entire body. Procreation, potency, fertility, and healthy sexual activity, imagination, pleasure of living, vitality, harmonious relationships and work with other people, action, tolerance, surrender, receiving and giving, all rely upon a strong sacral Chakra.

It resonates to the color orange and the note D. It carries the energies of imagination, desire, creativity and sexuality. It is the base of connecting to others. You will know when you are in balance in the sacral location as you'll be creatively expressive if you are artistic, a wordsmith, or expressive in your daily tasks including kid raising, your so on and job. You'll additionally be at ease with the sexuality in a means that's respectful of others and commands respect for yourself.

In case you don't love sex or are preoccupied with sex in a way, you might be out of stability in the sacral Chakra. Sacral Chakra have taken a battering through the years.

Lots of standard religions have tended towards connecting a lot of fear to sexuality and this worry has been carried down throughout the ages at various times society has possibly built on that or even moved away from it.

Of course, in present times we are becoming more and more connected to sexuality as self-expression and a full phrase of intimacy, the way we do currently have a lot of the way to visit and numerous individuals still wrestle with locating a method to have proper loving sexuality. Imagination too has been minimized and at times outlawed (Consider the Dark Ages during which all creative expression apart from religious art was totally banned).

Now we identify creativity as all expression of self, so the more confident we are, the more we express ourselves in all we do. Here are some few tasks to help you work towards balancing the Sacral Chakra.

Change your thinking about sexuality by reading books such as 'Reclaiming Goddess Sexuality' by Linda E. Savage.

Check out your own sexuality. The exploration can include treatment to unravel problems across the topic. Check out the creative side with mediums which excite you, words, colors, music.

Do not determine the end result, simply like the action of checking it out. Work with innovative Energy techniques to focus on power program and any harm that could be connected to or even influence on the Sacral Chakra. Developing the connection with this Chakra may be fun.

Knowing yourself, what is working and what is not in life is empowering, particularly as if you run into something that doesn't work. There are methods and also means of dealing with this and the outcome is often a significantly more enriched and loving lifestyle.

CHAPTER 7

SOLAR PLEXUS CHAKRA

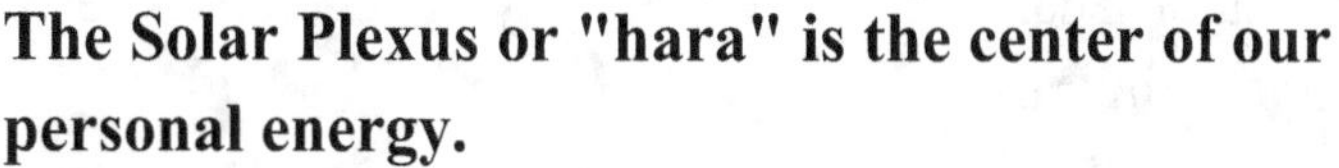

The Solar Plexus or "hara" is the center of our personal energy.

Mars, the planet related to private will and Pluto are the co-rulers of this 3rd Chakra. The problems of the 3rd Chakra have to do with control, power, our awareness of personal empowerment and also trusting our gut instincts.

A Chakra that is obstructed may manifest as a lack of the ability to make decisions, not needing to trust our own Instincts, and feelings of victimization or being manipulated. An overactive third Chakra could manifest as control problems, intimidation, rape, or even violence.

The key to curing the third Chakra is to understand how to use our power without damaging others. It's also very important to understand the way to let go of the anxiety of being in control.

Music could be a mean for opening the third Chakra since it's a non-verbal kind of communication that by-passes the cognitive thoughts and directly affects our deepest feelings.

Finding music that moves you, physically or emotionally is a mean of understanding the deeper feelings of despair and anger which are frequently trapped in this Chakra.

As these emotions are discovered and allowed saying, this Chakra can subsequently blossom and the energy that's been steered into command can now be re-routed to more satisfying types of self-expression and imagination. The third major Chakra of the entire body is generally known as the Manipura.

It is a Sanskrit word that means 'gem'. This Chakra is located in the solar navel plexus and the digestive system area which is also the site of intelligence. A solar plexus Chakra is related to self-esteem, energy, self-control, power and subject. People that have a solid 3rd Chakra have a tendency to display characteristics such as livelihood, internal power and self-confidence.

The organs and glands connected to the solar plexus Chakra are the gastrointestinal tract and the pancreas. That is the main reason one starts growing digestive issues with an imbalance in the solar plexus Chakra. Color – Gold and Silver are the colors of the Chakra.

So, if the Chakra is imbalanced, it's likely to get it back to equilibrium by focusing on yellowish or gold things such as gold and candle fires, by sporting more of yellow clothing and eating more yellow fruits and vegetables like carrots, squash and berry.

Fire is the element of the 3rd Chakra. But if there is too much of a heat from the Chakra area, a person may start developing troubles. It is likely to excite the 3rd Chakra by utilizing yoga. One needs to ensure that before performing Bikram yoga, the Chakra does require some stimulation. Anger is the emotion of this Chakra. An excessive third Chakra contributes to excessive focus on status, power and popularity, hate and anger. This may be subdued with passive backbends.

Cognitive and sight believing will be the sense for this Chakra. The wisdom can be seen here, and that's where some people now get a 'gut feeling' from while taking decisions. Wearing stones like tiger's eye, gold, peridot, chalcedony, yellow sapphire, yellow topaz or calcite helps stimulating and balancing the Chakra.

The yoga poses to help balance the 3rd Chakra are the half boat poses, spins, warrior and sun salutations.

An obstructed third Chakra

The health problems that arise from an obstructed third Chakra are nausea, diabetes, hypoglycemia, digestive issues, over-sexuality, depression, muscular cramps, eating disorders, skin ailments and problems in the spleen, kidneys, pancreas and nerve cells.

With numerous health problems arising out of a third Chakra that is obstructed, experts say that health complications may likewise result in individuals getting obsessed with power over everyone and everything. But when the Chakra is in equilibrium, the individual gains self-esteem spontaneity and develops self-identity.

They produce a power that originates in the middle of their human body from the solar plexus area which makes them feel as if they belonged everywhere. This contributes to the functioning of assimilation, metabolism and digestion of food. As people with a third strong Chakra are successful in their toes, specialists do agree that a variety of the greatest dancers have a potent Chakra.

Psychologically, the solar plexus relates to the feelings of individual energy inside the globe. Additionally, it assists in the development of a great ego. It's in touch with the adrenal glands as well as pancreas. The solar plexus Chakra pertains to the energy levels as well as digestion.

It is found in between the navel and the breastbone. When this Chakra is out of balance, it is usually a sign that one's stomach, liver or pancreas isn't working properly.

This is a Chakra that boosts psychic energy. It relates to a "second sight", the same energy that mediums work with. Launching this spectacle empowers a psychic reader to increase their psychic senses. This Chakra supports prophetic dreams and psychic intuition. It's from this particular ecosystem where we get "gut" feelings.

Essential Oils: Sandalwood, Chamomile, Rosemary, Frankincense, Rose, Myrrh, Rosewood.

Solar Plexus Chakra is your third Chakra and it's located above the belly button in the upper abdominal region, beneath the chest. Solar plexus Chakra governs our self-esteem, our sense of self confidence, and the development of power.

When the solar plexus Chakra is imbalanced, we encounter low self-esteem, self-image anxieties, fear of rejection, oversensitivity to criticism, and indecisiveness.

This really is about self-care, self-worth, assurance, and how we see ourselves compared to others. Are you afraid of failing? This is a typical third-party weakness.

Some of the body health problems that are related to the solar plexus are digestive problems, anemia, ulcers, diabetes, and liver diseases.

Mindfully consume. Chew your food nicely. Pamper yourself, take a great bath, or make a relaxing before foundation ritual. Make a meal and discuss it with your community.

Meditate on trusting yourself and appreciating who you are.

Crystal Correction: Golden Beryl is a gentle, orange-yellow-colored stone which directs will and enhances trust.

It's good for Chakra blockages. Placing this rock 2 inches above your navel will free your power center. For all those stressed by this particular Chakra, jade is as a way.

This calming stone decreases impulses towards various other individuals, and also allows to station our fires carefully.

This specific Chakra impacts your psychological body responsible for the self-esteem, self-identity, and purpose and the surrounding relationships. If you are experiencing mental problems and psychological stress issues that impede your way of living, even if they are manifested via indigestion, ulcers, fatigue and anxiety attacks, you have to get this Chakra in check.

Only some roads toward wellness are actually free from obstacles though we can get the aid of binaural beats not just to tune the Chakras or even make our wellness journey easier. It can additionally help us enhance some other places regarding life.

Solar plexus Chakra healing not just stems from metaphysical and mental adjustment, though. The body must participate in it as well. The food that we bring in issues as it nourishes and fuels the Chakras.

Be certain to include things like the following in the diet plan to provide the self-esteem an increase & foster self-love: grains- bread, cereal; and grain Spices- cumin, ginger, chamomile; cheese and dairy milk. You can likewise exercise the Chakra by enjoying belly dancing, using the hula hoop, and invite any person who's prepared to perform the twist.

While you heal & stimulate this specific Chakra, you will develop human relationships that are healthy, gain self-confidence and also, just simply celebrate life. We are capable of healing ourselves and strengthening the core being. You by yourself are able to unlock your full potential and make a sense of balance between your body and head.

It boils down to your openness and will to attain it. In order to keep the Chakras in tune and control a solar plexus Chakra healing, incorporate binaural beats to everyday exercise. They will help you get a heightened religious consciousness and actual physical power. The Solar Plexus Chakra is about your empowered state of being.

It is concerning being a secure and confident elf with no overriding others in the private choices for themselves. It is about realizing how you can be part of a team without sacrificing yourself or your sense of integrity. If you feel strong and confident that you dwell in the position to speak your mind, you also command respect from people in your way and attitude & treat others with respect.

Solar energy Plexus imbalance is something that has always existed. You will experience a tough time finding a society in history and especially the latest times which has not had issues based on power.

Dealing with these problems is actually a lifelong research of understanding and refinement, however, as a society, we are steadily coming along because of the rise of many smart instructors of real power like Martin Luther King, Mother Theresa and Nelson Mandela.

Here are few tasks which will help you balance the Solar Plexus Chakra: Spend a bit of time meditating linking to Solar Plexus Chakra listening to what it must be whole and empowered. Invest some time exploring the encounters of Control vs Empowerment. Think of a time when you have felt empowered.

Think of instances when you have experienced out of control situations. Just how did you behave? Just how have you dealt with yourself and others? Follow the threads of the understanding you are developing into areas of untapped energy and pain. Consider therapeutic labor to unravel places of damage and wounding. Do every day energy job therapies on yourself.

Work with innovative Energy Technicians to clean up and close down harm and interference impacting on daily life. Building the consciousness around Solar Plexus Chakra and the state of the Self in this specific place is a profoundly empowering procedure that is crucial. Naturally, what is available and suggested is simply the idea of the iceberg of what is obtainable in Consciousness Development because of this topic.

It is worth becoming dedicated to growing the understanding in this specific field and dealing with various resources and strategies to increase access to untapped energy in daily life.

CHAPTER 8
HEART CHAKRA

The Heart Chakra

The lungs and heart are dominated by the planet Venus. Venus represents what we value, what we are passionate about and also our capability to talk about love.

In addition, I assign a "higher" ruler ship of this fourth Chakra to the planet Neptune, since it's Neptune that symbolizes the practice of hammering our own identity and merging with our soul or divine love.

The 4th Chakra is the bridge between the higher and lower Chakras. It's been stated that our western civilization mostly relates to the difficulties of their first three Chakras: cash, gender and power.

As we psychologically understand the attachments of our first three Chakras, we can start to clearly perceive the expansive qualities of the higher Chakras. In the event of a blocked 4th Chakra, we may experience fears of never being loved, anxieties of giving and receiving affection or associations which are unfulfilling. The key to curing the heart Chakra is via the evolution of compassion, dedication, and a feeling of strong relationships with other people.

Music, the devotional singing type, can start the heart and reduce feelings of separation. Mixing sacred mantras from different religious traditions with dances of universal peace, simple circle dances, helps us let go of those walls that keep us different. They're also a very safe method of practicing the way of giving and receiving unconditional love.

The 4th Chakra is situated in the center of the torso behind the breastbone. This is the centerstage of connection, empathy, retrieval, compassion, affinity for others and self. The element connected to the Chakra is atmosphere.

Heart Chakra Color

The relevant colors for the heart Chakra are gold, green and pink.

These colors are due to the "shift in the psychic energies of this evolving heart". Throughout our productive adulthood years, it should be regarded as pink, the integration of the white (function) color of the crown and the red (fire) color of the first melody.

This is a result of advices we grew up with: it's far better to give than receive, and we have to care for everyone else first, because caring for ourselves is "egotistical". The reality, in fact, is that if we don't love and care for ourselves, we will never have love to give to somebody else. We live on the inside. The love we give ourselves fixes the norm for a healthy relationship, one where we get up to, we supply.

Everybody in this world is here to experience development, roughing their elbows up, falling down so that they could get up. That is exactly what we came for. What we could call mistakes are lessons to move beyond and it is no one's obligation to protect someone else. Parents might have a tricky time with this.

The heart Chakra is responsible for our fantasies and desires. At the middle, down the arms and out of the hands as healing energy flows, renewable energy does.

I have seen debilitating energy when creativity has been squelched. It physically controls lungs and the heart and also modulates the thymus. When out of balance, there's a risk for heart issues and immune deficiencies.

The Heart Chakra is situated at the middle of your torso, between your shoulder blades. It is linked to our universal mind. Emotionally, it pertains to honesty and love. An individual may lack kindness and compassion.

This is the Chakra relating to connection. It affects the way you're feeling amongst others. Additionally, it affects your feelings of self and self-worth.

We're all about love, forgiveness, compassion, unconditional love, acceptance from people that are different from us. An under-active heart Chakra will manifest as feeling unloved, seeking love other than fostering racism and self-love.

Some disorders related with the heart Chakra are breast cancer, cardiovascular disease, respiratory problems, and upper back pain. Suggestions for the heart Chakra: Lead through example. Eat more sour greens (watercress, kale, arugula, bok choy). Keep a gratitude journal. This really is the heart Chakra and its role is self-explanatory. This is the celestial world of spiritual growth, high ideals, love, and resilience.

A heart Chakra that is congested makes us critical of both ourselves and others. In such condition, we find it difficult to open ourselves up to possibilities required for friendship and love. Conversely, if our heart is too big, we might attempt to do the impossible, trying to take on the weight of earth.

Crystal Correction: The green jasper helps us feel secure to open up and show ourselves. This eases joyful and honest communication. To get a heart with no bounds, it's advisable you try peridot. This pastel rock recharges us. Peridot allows us to be unsacrificial and sympathetic.

Amber can be helpful within this capacity. Beings with effective heart Chakras have much love, might have empathy for others, compassion, understanding, forgiveness, team consciousness, contentment, acceptance, peace, typically breathe deeply with a slow rhythm, have powerful lungs, proper heart, and fresh blood flow, hardly ever experiencing bronchial or respiratory ailments; as the lungs belong to the air component, this indicates an instant connection with the respiratory system. Getting rid of blockages to the heart Chakra, can likewise help preventing coronary issues.

The heart Chakra additionally governs the arms, hands, top back, shoulders, and rib cage. The touch sensation is actually governed by the heart Chakra.

Heart Chakra Healing

The Heart Chakra is the center of the whole Human Energy System. Whenever we continue bringing ourselves back again to heart-centered status, the system restores to its optimum aligned condition and the complete program works brilliantly. In case you work with Matrix Technicians, it shifts and holds a lot more easily.

It is when the system product is extremely well-aimed that you are quicker in aligning with the life you picked, the partner, cash, the soul phrase etc. Some call it manifesting, I call it alignment - meaning you are aligning with life as it supports the purpose for being here - as it supports you effectively.

The 4th Chakra, located at the actual center of the breast cage or chest, is connoted by the Anahata Mandala which literally means "unstruck sound."

It is also symbolized with four-legged mammals. The lower 3 Chakras connect to egoic power and the greater 3 Chakras connect to the greater self-energy and the source of consciousness.

The heart Chakra is the center point where these two realms converge. It provides a bridge between the ego and the greater self (spirit). If the Chakra needs healing, the physical diseases will affect the lungs, blood circulation or cause heart issues. We might feel rejected, uncared for, unappreciated, unloved, and might play the martyr role.

Love provided outward always includes a tether to something expected back in return. Thus, we fail in personal human relationships, personal friendships, and wind up feeling very lonely and disconnected in life.

Often when the Chakra is blocked, this is a consequence of abandonment as kids and then this exact same behavioral construct repeats itself throughout life until we are able to forgive.

With forgiveness comes acceptance. And it frees us from the bondage of loneliness. Mainly through the action of forgiving people who trespass against us very profoundly could the heart Chakra be freed, and the real power released.

If the Chakra is balanced, we'll be having compassion towards every human being and can loving everybody unconditionally.

We like and accept living unconditionally, regardless of what scenario or challenge life brings to us. This is referred to as living in the Now. Our lives take on a meaning that is new since we understand the truth behind the aphorism "You have to give, in order to receive."

As a result, we ultimately become pursuers, activists, and philanthropists of altruistic endeavors. Supposing we are not assisting others in a way, we are just not keen on spending the time and effort to get it done. A Counselor could suggest you on the right resources and modalities for healing the heart Chakra.

Essential oils and the flowers are all green flowers or yellow flowers, rose geranium, jasmine, neroli, tea tree, peppermint, patchouli, ylang-ylang, pinewood, clover, grass rose oil. The crystals for healing are: emerald, jade, rose quartz, eco-friendly aventurine, agate, malachite, tourmaline, and dioptase.

So how can you begin aligning with the heart Chakra? You will find so many levels of this particular work, you can make use of electricity work (working with the Chakras) you can make use of mental labor (imagining going into the heart and concentrating on the love you do have for someone).

Right here I write about a powerful and simple Heart Alignment Process which I have been dealing with and teaching individuals to work with for numerous years. Picture the Heart Chakra in case it really works for you, view it as a lovely spinning ball of light. In the center, an outstanding point of light, such as a star, eternal ever-present, absolute.

Move into the light, be still and present in there, this is you, it is yours, it is sacred and absolute and you are aligning with it forever. Invest some time in this each day, go back to it throughout the day. While you carry on and do this procedure, you will find it becomes much easier and you will be able to remain in your heart center much more readily.

Even though that physical exercise appears easy, based on the attention you place towards dealing with it, over time it may become incredibly effective, especially in case you invest time concentrating on and moving into the gorgeous sacred lighting of the center. Once you perfect this exercise, you will find much more you can work with to go deeper into this particular work.

You will find that the more you work with the Chakra in this fashion, the more you can 'self-align' to an important degree. The heart Chakras is situated in the center of the chest. It vibrates to the colors green and rose pink and also the musical note F. The Chakra is about the state of love. All Love, like is actually a state of being, it is a vibration.

It is something we think in conjunction with the family, friends, lovers, kids, the planet and I am certain you can think of more. Through hurtful happenings such as neglectful or abusive childhoods & relationships, folks close the hearts off in an attempt to desist from pain once again.

Nevertheless, everything this does is block the flow of love itself (which will be a great portion of relationships), the agonizing experiences have a tendency to continue in different ways.

Here are a few tasks which that will help you bring peace, balance, and healing to your heart Chakra: Journaling (write down the things/people trigger love responses within you, take the time you might discover that you have problems thinking of anything, therefore think of small things, a flower or a bird). Spend time each day thinking of and writing about love which is actually triggered. Strong in the heart of everyone's center is a divine spark of light.

Tune into your own light and then travel deep into it, feeling the love and peace there, then concentrate on someone else's light and do exactly the same. Focus on the light of a person you like and then simply if you feel positive with the experience, concentrate on someone you do not like. Feel their Inner Light rather compared to their character. Meditate on the heart Chakra.

Do everyday energy therapies on yourself. Get an Auric Technician to work with so they can focus on your system shutting down harm and cleaning up interference so that the Chakra is actually operating nicely. Explore the ways in which you may have disconnected from love, life, folks, the planet.

Think about finding an excellent therapist or therapeutic team to work with any wounding you might have uncovered. Love is such an important gas for human life. deepening the consciousness around the connection with love and the state of the Chakra could really shift you out of many years of blocked and hurting patterns of thought and behavior.

CHAPTER 9
THROAT CHAKRA

The Throat Chakra

The fifth Chakra, situated in the throat region is regulated by Mercury, the planet representing all kinds of communicating and Chiron, representing the mentor/teacher archetype.

It's throughout the fifth Chakra we build personal reflection and the capacity to create our own reality. In the event the Chakra is blocked, we may have anxiety of speaking up for ourselves. It could also be hard to express our requirements or the feelings we experience originating from the heart Chakra.

Another frequent manifestation of an obstructed fifth Chakra is disbelief in our capacity to design our own lives how we've imagined. When we mature with no voice based on decisions that were being made for us, we might cease to believe in the ability of our free will or voice. Fixing the 5th Chakra is imperative if we wish to open into the instinctive awareness that comes in the sixth and seventh Chakras.

When the Chakra is blocked, we might be too psychological rather than amenable to the delicate intuitive advice that's always being channeled via the bigger centers. Concerning healing modalities, singing is just one of the most effective methods for opening the Chakra.

Since most individuals with fifth Chakra blockages have "lost their voice", the best way to regain our voice would be to vibrate it with noise! Chanting mantras that are sacred such as OM can also be valuable, as OM is viewed as the basic or primordial sound of this world.

When we chant OM, we ultimately align ourselves with all the creative sound that's considered to attract all stuff form into presence. The purpose of the 5th Chakra is "the capability to define ourselves out of the entire world". This isn't necessarily easy to accomplish since the energy that's behind this saying is certainty and certainty comes out from a sense of worth and value.

Unworthiness and invalidation are all energies that obstruct the Chakra. Perhaps in this life or past, it wasn't feasible to speak the truth for fear of persecution, punishment or even death. This energy might be irrational in this present lifetime but the fears it arouses are extremely genuine and shut down that communicating center.

Another energy that blocks the 5th Chakra is responsible for estimating, censoring or swallowing the phrases in order to be approved by the person that you're speaking to if that is eventually great for you or not. I am not speaking about being socially okay I am speaking about not being truthful to yourself in order to eventually become "okay" with someone else or group of individuals.

The 5th Chakra is the engine vehicle for discharging and processing emotion. "Discussing it" is a great explanation of talking through your emotions, which releases them in the physical body. The Yang or incoming purpose of the 5th Chakra is about expressing. Yin's purpose or the open minded of the 5th Chakra is responsible for getting information.

The color associated with this Chakra is gloomy. The 5th Chakra is the bridge between the elemental decreased four Chakras and believed (sixth Chakra) and soul (seventh Chakra). The 5th Chakra is the ether or space where the four elements exist. At this level (neck), we experience the standard of distance.

This is the attribute of the element of ether. Clairaudience is the ability of the Chakra that enables you to receive messages in the kind of thoughts from other frequency or realm as it is considered to be a channel. The throat Chakra relates to creativity, communication, and personal development.

Situated at the upper part of the throat, the throat Chakra rules the nose, thyroid, eyes, ears, and mouth area. This Chakra correlates into the expression of one's emotions. When open, it assists in communicating with others both psychically and verbally. In addition, this is the

Chakra of rationale and logic. When closed, one may have creative blocks, sore throats, and miscommunications.

Essential Oils: Bergamot and Basil, Peppermint, Spearmint, Chamomile

The 5th Chakra is found in the neck, ears and throat. The Chakra governs our ability to effectively communicate as well as to listen and understand others. When it is out of equilibrium, an individual can have trouble expressing themselves, repress feelings and experience poor learning ability.

Other symptoms of an imbalance are doubt, habitual lying, feelings of fear etc.

Throat Chakra (Shoulders, colon, thyroid, neck)

Here we reflect on our capacity to go to substance attachments, or items that no longer serve us. This Chakra gets us connected to our spirit and represents our ability to effectively communicate with other people, our authentic voice.

Several the health problems that are related to this Chakra are esophageal cancer, thyroid problems, chronic sore throat, and shoulder and neck pain. Sing, engage in drama (the performance Kind, not the energy-sucking workplace type) and compose. Meditate while focusing on your breath. Express what you stand for to other people.

It's represented by the circadian rhythm and light. Many psychological illnesses are manifested here: obstructed believing, obsessive compulsive behaviors, constantly reliant on others for advice, and inadequate self-awareness. Tap into your intuition. Switch off the Electronics and sit in silence. Listen to your inner voice. Practice this for 20 minutes daily.

Eat seasonally and locally and use fresh Spices and herbs in cooking. Cut down caffeine and alcohol.

It's situated at the lower part of the throat. When this Chakra is balanced, we talk honestly. Sodalite crystal is a stunning navy rock that helps to ease a throat that is constricted.

This crystal promises clarity and courage. On the other hand, people who have a 5th Chakra have to speak the truth quietly. Amber can be helpful within this capacity. This Chakra gives the ability to communicate with other people and diffuse ideas. This particular Chakra has to do with imagination and taking the proper choices.

To enjoy the healing advantages of the Chakra, endeavor to focus on confidence and sharing ideas. You need to let your imagination explore and think of exciting ideas and terminologies. Blockage in this Chakra can result in stunted creativity and make someone incredibly introvert.

A rich sound of one's voice is actually the sound of a great throat Chakra. One who breathes readily, won't experience any throat or tonsils inflammations. And the influence impact on the larynx, and vocal cords the throat Chakra likewise could impact the esophagus, throat, tongue, skin, gums, vertebrae in jaw, teeth, mouth, hands, the shoulders & windpipe, arms and the neck.

It regulates the thyroid and parathyroid glands - which together command suitable metabolism of minerals, protein, calcium, water, fat, carbohydrates and the central nervous system.

It rules truth inspiration, musical abilities, communication, perceptions, creative expression of speech, righteous (right-use-of-will) discrimination, publishing and the arts, wisdom, knowledge, truths, reliability, honesty, loyalty, peace kindness.

Additional emotional connections to this particular Chakra connect to dynamic will, creativity, acknowledgment and self-support, ability to go by one's aspiration.

If the throat Chakra isn't healthy one could suffer from lassitude or nervousness, throat soreness, speech defects, tonsillitis.), periodontal or dental issues, problems with the shoulder and neck pain, stiffness in the shoulders and neck, under-active or overactive thyroids, shyness, failure to express oneself.

The Throat Chakra as The Voice In The World - this particular Chakra is about interaction, both receiving and giving.

It is about the communication you get and just how you interpret it. A lot of females that I've worked with have had long-term issues with their throats. They have' kept their peace' in relationships, meaning they haven't reported the elements they intend to point out and also have gone without as a result.

Even though this does occur in males too, by far females have shown to be probably the strongest carriers of this condition. It manifests as repeated clearing of the throat or coughing, a raspy throat or altered speech like an extremely gentle or high-pitched throat like a kid.

I've additionally viewed the frequently startlingly fast recovery of the cases once they are urged to speak out about just who they are and the things they select in their lives and whenever they begin to check out and uncover the numerous things they have kept secret inside.

Additionally, there are individuals who talk way too loudly as they believe they are never heard. These folks likewise feel unheard and the result is speaking louder and louder.

If somebody counter acts what they are saying, this will make them think they are not being understood so that they frequently speak louder and are hostile.

These problems will make them feel unloved, unheard, misunderstood, and lonely. These and other problems of the Chakra have to be dealt with so you can use a loving, joy-filled lifestyle.

Here are a few approaches of dealing together with your throat Chakra: Read books on communication and self-expression. Find out about communication of relationships. Study yummy power to communicate with other people.

Are you sincere, real, kind, mild, respectful? Do you think you are in a position to clearly communicate everything you select for yourself or what you believe when it differs with other opinions? Do you think you are capable to hear other's opinions without overreacting? Start up a log and truly voice the deepest truths including those things you have never said out loud.

When you have a while to yourself, stand in the comfort of your home and express some things you like about yourself, list things about yourself you are feeling shame near or fear about.

Talk these items out loud and observe just how easy/difficult you think it is to do that. Should you learn you do struggle profoundly with communication and self-expression, think about locating a good therapeutic team or therapist to work within this specific place.

Begin dealing with an innovative Auric Technician who'll go deeper into the system and locate harm, interference, and wiring which will be repaired so that the product is supporting the choice for excellent, empowered living.

A throat Chakra is an incredible tool when working. It enables you to confidently and fully express the Sacred Truth of who you are on the planet and in all elements of life.

Its functioning will totally depend upon the amount of consciousness in the wellbeing and any wounding and damage you might have in this specific area. Committing to a deepening recognition of the healing and this Chakra of the relationship with it is going to alter everyday living.

CHAPTER 10
THIRD EYE CHAKRA

This Chakra is located at the middle of the forehead is co-ruled by the Moon and Sunlight.

The 6th Chakra is related to our high mental skills of intuition, introspection, self-examination, and perception. Traditionally, the sixth Chakra is viewed as having two sticks.

The moon rod, situated Medulla, is where we get the "breath of god" or universal energy. The sunlight or busy rod situated in the third eye is where we stock this universal energy via the vehicle of our own identity.

A Chakra that is obstructed may manifest as anxiety of appearing inside ourselves, refusal to learn from life adventures, anxiety about using our instinctive skills, or even the inability to get inner guidance.

Physical symptoms may include depression, migraines, stress, and learning disabilities. Among the best ways to start the 6th Chakra is by visualization, meditation, and obtaining the imaginal world through dreamwork.

This opening could be eased by music which arouses the creativity and leads us to the world of non-ordinary insights. We have access to lots of available CDs that assist the mind to get deeper conditions of delta, alpha, and theta consciousness which are otherwise just generated via meditation practices.

The 6th Chakra is referred to as the Third Eye and may be found in the center of the head, behind the eyes and between the ears.

This is the centerstage of thought, intuition, ingenuity, inspiration and clairvoyance. Thought is where everything starts, the "primary cause". Everything that we see in our world began in our bodies as thought.

The 6th Chakra is the inner control center. We can utilize this Chakra to understand what, by making use of our imagination, we would like to encounter.

This Chakra is the location where we can detect what is happening in our lives with neutrality. If you take consciousness or your attention into the sixth Chakra, you'll observe that you aren't at the emotion of the lower Chakra and may discover what is happening. You might be the observer and, with neutrality, you can view and act clearly.

Within my practice, we created a room within our sixth Chakras known as our "Center of Head Room". It's the place where we navigate clairvoyantly. If you're not interested in clairvoyance, the middle of the mind is a stunning place to make an inner sanctuary for prayer and meditation.

The subject of moving into your inner sanctuary in order to communicate is valuable in my own opinion. Make it somewhere you like to be, where you are fed and nurtured.

Energy that blocks the 6th Chakra is your view that imagination is counterproductive to achievement and may be a waste of time. This sort of information not only blocks the potent expression of the sixth Chakra, but it may include guilt and self-judgment for indulging in "daydreaming". The color corresponding with the 6th Chakra is Indigo. The 3rd eye Chakra fosters the practice of abstract thoughts.

Additionally, it allows us to experience the spirit world. It is the center of intuition and awareness. The Third Eye relates to your eyes, pituitary gland and sinuses. This Chakra relates to the capacity of visualizing and proceeding information. Emotionally, the 3rd eye Chakra signifies acceptance and tolerance. At the same time, the 3rd Chakra is the energy that drives us.

When available, this Chakra enables us to manifest our needs and be responsible for our decisions. Concerning psychic abilities, the third eye encompasses how we understand things, this includes the feelings of others and emotion. Additionally, it enables us to maximize our extra sensory perception.

For the psychic reader, the 3rd eye Chakra lets them view the larger image of things with a skill known as clairvoyance. This is the capacity to find pictures in your mind's eye.

Essential Oils: Patchouli, Cypress and Juniper, Sandalwood, Clary Sage, Vetiver,

The 3rd Eye Chakra is your sixth Chakra and it is situated on the forehead between the eyebrows. The Chakra governs our ability to use common sense, spirituality, intellect, wisdom, translate dreams and intuition.

When it is out of equilibrium, one may lack instinct, have sleep difficulties, experience common sense trouble, be forgetful, and suffer from confusion. Most know this energy center between the brows as the third eye.

If in equilibrium, this Chakra gives us the capability to show our innate psychic capacity. But we limit ourselves to unproven facts when it is obstructed. This also leads to thinking that is stiff and disrupted joy.

If we're too open, we may be disconnected from the physical world - an inability to close the eye that is psychic. If we dream, we must wake up.

Correction: A moonstone located on the brow center Chakra clears the issues that blindfolded our intuition and directly opens our mind thus embracing personal development, because moonstone is connected to cycles of change. This helps us tune in to stream, welcoming spontaneity and discharging rigidity.

With an open eye, blue lace agate is required. This sky-blue crystal stone helps clearing out the mess of distraction and sharpens our attention.

The Brow Chakra as The Vision

The Brow Chakra is actually situated on the forehead between the eyebrows.

The color related to it is deep dark indigo, a lovely purple/blue. It sparkles with light, particularly when active and healthy. It resonates with the note A. Tuning into this Chakra is all about tuning in the Inner Vision.

This Chakra relates to the way you see the planet. Additionally, it provides you with visions in the waking and dreaming state. All too frequently family history, previous living trauma, and other interferences have meant that the individual has attempted to block off this Chakra in an attempt to desist from seeing what is developing.

Naturally, that doesn't prevent terrible things from happening but does develop a sort of relief for the person, therefore they are inclined to help keep it there. This additionally causes a lot of troubles, as you are setting up a scenario in which you can 'see less' of what took place in your life. Consider when you hated everything you had been seeing in your childhood, so you cut out the eyes.

You probably won't be seeing what is happening, though you will nonetheless be experiencing it in some other ways and at exactly the same time tripping over everything since you would be oblivious.

Effectively, blocking the brow Chakra (or some other Chakra) has exactly the same outcome. Activities for balancing and healing with the brow Chakra: take a look at the ways in which you perceive the planet and the places surrounding you.

Is this perception giving you a positive feeling? Can you really feel safe? If not, realize that the way you 'see' the earth is just how you will experience it and therefore, shifting the focus to a happier, better type of trust, will result in a much better experience. Meditate on the brow Chakra speaking to it, asking concerns and listening for info about what it must be balanced and healthy.

Ask your 3rd eye to trigger and get stronger, wider open as you would like to feel the truth of everything you see. Gather scarves of various (single) colors and one at a time, tie them round the brow. Sit with every color and tune into the sensations, thoughts, energies and other subtleties they provide.

Believe the pulls and stretches on the brow as you wear the various styles. Have a dream journal, writing down the dreams exploring their messages and symbolism for you. Do everyday Energy therapies on yourself. Connect with an innovative Auric Technician so they can work with the computer clearing it of interference, repairing and rewiring any harm.

Decelerate and see your perception of the planet. Perception is crucial to the experience, so be sure the perception isn't warped and dim. If It is, think about checking out with a therapist to uncover and unravel the harm to ensure that you can restore notions to the Conscious Choice. It is the seat of the belief. Life choices and knowledge are greatly formed by the belief.

To deepen the Consciousness around this Chakra and your weaknesses and strengths of this specific place can provide big shifts in life.

Third eye (between the pineal gland, eyebrows, eyes) - The Chakra relates to your instinct, intellect, and dreaming. It's represented by circadian rhythm and light.

Many psychological illnesses are manifested here: obstructed believing, obsessive compulsive behaviors, constantly reliant on others for advice, and inadequate self-awareness.

Hints for the sixth Chakra:

Tap into your intuition. Switch off the electronics and sit in quiet. Listen to your inner voice. Practice this for 20 minutes daily. Eat seasonal and local foods and use fresh spices and herbs when cooking. Cut down the caffeine and alcohol.

CHAPTER 11
CROWN CHAKRA

Last, we hit the seventh Chakra, located in the very top or crown of the head. This crown Chakra is seen as another stage of entrance of energy and reflects our relationship with universal comprehension. I connect the Chakra using the planet Uranus, since its Uranus which reflects the universal current of energy that calms mind, body and soul.

In the Vedic standpoint of India, Uranus signifies the kundalini energy which resides in the lower part of the spine from the first Chakra.

As we wake up and open all the interrelated kundalini energies, we climb up the backbone and trigger the seventh Chakra, resulting in illumination or enlightenment. Many people experience this when having an orgasm because the kundalini moves with the lower Chakras and activating the crown Chakra.

The main reason we go to sleep is that we aren't used to directing that much energy at the greater centers, so we wind up shutting down, or even going unconscious. When we have blockages in the seventh Chakra, this could manifest as reduced life force, disbelief the ability to find enjoyment in the world, or a feeling of disconnection from our direction or meaning in life.

The intriguing thing about the seventh Chakra is that it's the polar opposite of the very first loaf so we can open it from "above" or "below". Pranayama or breathing techniques help open the seventh Chakra by enlarging our capability to channel energy through the top of the head. As we enlarge our capability to channel energy, we could withstand more aliveness going through our bodies with no immunity.

As we open the lower Chakras through sound and movement, we reduce the resistance we need to be livelier and discharge the kundalini energy that's dormant at the lower part of the spine. To put it differently, opening the higher Chakras doesn't necessarily mean that we have to dismiss or "transcend" the lower Chakras as some customs would have us think.

Instead, it demands that we work on establishing the whole chaotic field so that we gain the potential to experience higher states of awareness at an embodied way. The Seventh Chakra or the Crown Center sits flat on the mind's surface and is the path to the spirit. The Chakra is the center where we understand the divine truth, the "I AM" and where we get inspiration, instinct, and advice.

It may be described as "The psychics hub" for increased comprehension, it receives the spiritual energies and advice required to trigger our goal. It includes the capability to live our celestial identity by expressing intention, along with the yin capacity to take part in energies critical to feeding our religious character. As beings, Chakras include information from this lifetime in addition.

There are some kinds of energy which I see impeding the Chakra; one must do with beliefs and principles and another must do with value. The spiritual kind of energy can reveal that we, as individuals, can't receive advice straight. A variety of the energy could be quite stern.

Another energy handling value is the understanding that we are celestial beings and the and we have a birthright to receive inspiration and advices. Information is coming continuously but unless we're accepting and are aware of it we won't receive it. How many times do we get a reply to a request for help and question it or talk ourselves out of it entirely? We do not think we deserve it.

The simple reality is that we are psychic although answers come to folks who are spiritual. The expression "psychic" is a Greek word and it just means "of the Spirit". Since we exist, we are connected; we don't need to fulfill with some other criteria and we have to trust inspiration and advice.

The Crown Chakra is the center of the frequency of energy vibration. The color associated with this Chakra is purple. Essential Oils: Lavender, Rose and Sandalwood, Cedarwood, Frankincense, Jasmine,

The7th Chakra is located at the peak of the head and helps us connect and communicate with the Spirit. Once this Chakra is out of balance you might feel like you are lacking creativity and are emotionally pumped.

You may turn out to be very materialistic, trapped in previous pain and anxious about the future. Focusing on material possessions may be your way to sense full. Here are simple ways you may use aromatherapy to help balance your mind.

- Take a bath or shower with products made with the essential oils which are tuned to the specific Chakra.

- Use a tissue with few drops of the desirable essential oil and breathe deeply focusing on equilibrium.

- Burn incense during meditation.

- Wear clothes or jewelry of this color corresponding to the Chakra while you concentrate on creating harmony and balance.

Crown Chakra (Pituitary gland, cerebral cortex)

The seventh Chakra is the farthest, removed from the body and material things.

It is our spirituality, belief in divine power and the source of hope and faith. Emotional illnesses of this Chakra include feeling lost, without a goal in life, depression, schizophrenia and suicidal thoughts. Take the time to "cleanse" your mind, same as you don't think twice about cleaning your dirty clothes. Push out the negative thoughts and breathe in positive ones.

Exercise your spirituality: church, praying, spells, meditation. Reflect on why you are thankful for in life. Words aren't enough to express the capacity of this Chakra. It represents enlightenment. Even though balancing the Chakra can't make us a Buddha, it will certainly take us to peaks of bliss and help us connect with the purpose of our life. You are far from alone, if you are blocked here.

We might be confused about our career when blocked and lack calmness that was rapturous, that was lasting. For maximum results at balancing this Chakra, we must ensure the wellbeing of our prior Chakras. If you don't dislike stability and joy, possessing this particular Chakra is an issue.

We can communicate with the sorrowful and cynic. Otherwise we are trapped in our own mind which can get pretty lonely. The clear quartz is a perfect healer for a lot of Chakras and particularly useful for opening a closed crown Chakra. Due to the Chakra's place, the crystal chosen should be modest enough to rest on the head.

This stone offers clarity of purpose and makes it possible to see the meaning. It guides us to comprehend and live with truths. For all those with an open crown Chakra, hematite is perfect. By drawing attention, this stone helps us fulfill our own earthly needs.

Once again there's a bit of controversy about which color is best related to this particular Chakra point, though all of it depends on what resonates inside the Chakra and energy fields.

Probably the common crystals for this particular Chakra point are: Prehnite, Lapis Lazuli, Sugilite, Fluorite, Amethyst, and Iolite. In order to eliminate a Chakra blockage at this stage, hold Fluorite on the side of the Chakra and Prehnite within four inches of the Chakra.

Turn clockwise to remove the blockages. Remember to clean the crystal completely later to eliminate any dynamic buildup which has built upon the crystal. For a full energy flow, lie down and put 2 Amethyst crystals, on each side of the Chakra point and one on the region for fifteen minutes. It will improve the power for a far more powerful flow.

The Crown Chakra as The Brilliant Mind

This Chakra is situated in addition to the head, towards the front side. It resonates to bright purple and vibrates to the musical note B. It is mainly about the intellect and linking to Higher Consciousness and also the Spirit World.

This is exactly where the balance of spiritual connection and intellect (which is restricted to white and black, on and off, yes and no concepts) and infinity are actually well balanced.

We have all seen or even found out about individuals who block out mysticism and spirituality (as an example) in any way The worry and hysteria in a way of interaction are so frequently apparent. This is a good example of the Crown Chakra out of balance.

Intellect is very important, nonetheless, it may become extremely enticing to just concentrate on intellect. It is white and black; it creates a feeling of certainty and safety. It could be extremely appealing to shift into the emphasis of that white and black world, rejecting something that doesn't fit into it.

This is, itself, delusional, because as we know, the incredible Universe we live in is white and black. It is likewise easy to be out of balance with an over-reliance on the religious encounter, excluding the intellect.

This could lead to individuals who think whatever comes the way psychically - not what happens spiritually is coming from Light-based intelligence. There's Consciousness in the Spirit World which enjoys chaos and destruction.

For instance, the individual that receives signs that points them to a place they wish they were - such as jumping from one potentially terrible connection to the next - disregarding that their signs are frequently steering them in the incorrect direction? The balance of intellect and humility is an effective force so ensuring this particular life balance is advisable.

Tasks that can help balance the crown Chakra: if you are psychically active, focus on the quality of the messages you are getting.

Look at patterns of disaster in life (for instance, are you one of those individuals that keeps helping toxic peoplein your life?). Do you come out of those interactions mindful? Explore principles that increase your understanding of the Universe.

Hawkins Research with Advanced Energy Technicians, individuals that succeed in the power system of the Universe and comprehend and contend with Interfering Consciousness which strives to eliminate rather than produce. Observe your own balance of intellectual and psychic flow.

Think about how well it really works for you. Check the sources. The Crown Chakra truly links you into the Spirit World and psychic flow, however, it should be purposely handled both at the amount of intellect and the flow of outside consciousness.

Building the consciousness across the various channels of info flowing inwards and just how you sort and handle life via the Crown Chakra can result in some astonishing realizations and reclaiming of the territory of your daily life.

PART 3
HEALING YOUR
CHAKRA

CHAPTER 12
FOODS THAT HELP WITH HEALING

A nicely balanced body is created by using a balanced diet, by well-balanced surroundings and comprehension of the need to balance the 7 Chakras with each other.

Only in presence of stability from within and without, do we find true bliss, or parts of the ego, or Chakras are in equilibrium or harmony. It's when all seven Chakras are in equilibrium that we may reach our highest self. It's also the nutritious balance of these Chakras that relates and balances both our soul and lifestyle that is spiritual.

All seven Chakras should keep alignment and be cared for. These 7 tips below will aid balance and you can start to heal your seven Chakras. We must eliminate negative energy and foods out of our bodies. This measure involves replacing up over processed foods in our daily diet using fresh, live foods.

Making sure you drink a lot of tepid and purified water, jointly with foods that are organic helps to provide the section of the balance.

We must remove all forms of unwanted thinking from our head as far as possible. Many think negatively, talk negatively to themselves and others and hold grudges. A person must begin to alter this to replace those negative thoughts, emotions and activities with positive ones.

Keep a journal entry of every negative thought that springs to your mind, write it down, cross it out, then write a connection. You will discover in the forthcoming weeks considerably more favorable energy from the inside.

Avoid people who speak and behave negatively. Until you are balanced you may decide to avoid them however.

You need to modify negative behaviors, as far as you can and make room for positive energy. This may imply to connect to the community or surroundings rather than watching a violent film. Or it could mean starting a relaxing hobby that gives you quiet time. Attempt to promote recovery from the inside. This might be a spiritual movement for a few, and it might be a trip for others.

Attempt to provide a religious and harmonic balance on your religious life and outlook towards other men and women. Some people may utilize tapes with sound that is gentle or visualizations while others may prefer to sit down on the grass every day and listen to other nature sounds. Whichever you choose, make it a daily habit of 15 to 30 minutes. Schedule it at the beginning, until it becomes normality.

Look at your body with an exercise that is refreshing. This does not mean you have to take up workout or body building for lengthy amounts of time every day. An easy walk of 15 or 20 minutes should be enough. Have a type of yoga exercise like mild or Kundalini yoga, Pilates or hatha yoga ballet.

These both encourage wellness, energy, Chakra circulation and balance and rejuvenate the adrenal glands. Some people discover that fasting each week helps. You might discover that doing a natural or a colon cleansing a couple of times per year could help.

This may encourage energy in addition to poisonous build from waste and contamination to be taken out of your system. Bathe daily. Maintain the inside of yourself and also the exterior of yourself clean for great balance.

Establish limits to the quantity of work you do. Work smarter, not harder. Learn to manage your money. Take out some time to unwind and reflect.

Establish limits with yourself and other people. Sleep is known as unintentional meditation. It is the right time for the body to shut down balance and external stimulation. Be certain that you get good and enough sleep.

When you operate on the Chakras, you're going to be directly affecting that portion of your own life, as an instance, finances, sex life, self-esteem, compassion, stating, intuition and spirituality. Once your Chakras are balanced, then your life will feel balanced.

Each Chakra is important for a normal functioning of the body in line with the Chakra healing convention. Many powerful tools may impact the vibration of Chakras, and that's where balancing of Chakra comes to play.

Chakra stones, the individual voice, songs, chants, mantras and Chakra meditation contribute to bring the frequency of the Chakras back into appropriate vibrational alignment.

The root Chakra is heavily influenced by the ruby, hematite, onyx, or garnet gemstones. During dentistry recovery, a professional can utilize one or all these Chakra rocks to wash your root Chakra and bring it into balance.

Energy recovery helps balance the seven Chakras. It's quite typical in the modern world with hectic schedules, poor diets and lack of sleep to have our Chakras unbalanced. I'd guess that most individuals don't even understand what it feels like to get their own Chakras in equilibrium.

Energy recovery will permit you to get back in contact with your body. Chakra energy recovery will also allow you to feel balanced, complete and provide a general sense of wellness. Make sure the Chakra energy recovery technique feels appropriate for you and you're familiar with it.

The Chakra energy recovery process I will discuss now involves using diamonds. Typically, the bead will possess the same color as the Chakra is supposed to balance. This technique could be performed one Chakra at a time or seven Chakras simultaneously. This may be quite beneficial if you understand you have a specific charm from equilibrium.

First start with a great cleansing of those Chakras. Have a rock such as black obsidian for your cleanup procedure. This rock is known to extract the negative energy that could be lodged on your mind. Set the stone on your writing hand and then transfer it on the Chakra to be cleansed in a counterclockwise motion.

As you're doing so, picture in the eye of your mind on the negative energies coming out and being absorbed into the rock. You ought to begin with the root Chakra and proceed one Chakra at a time.

You will observe that certain Chakras will require more cleanup than others. Once you believe the Chakras are cleansed, now it's time to proceed to putting the rocks along with the Chakra energy recovery.

Assuming you will do the Chakra energy recovery together for all of the Chakras, begin by putting the corresponding bead on each one. You need to work from the root. It can be helpful to have someone help set the diamonds on you.

A few examples of the stones I use for every corresponding Chakra are as follows.

In Chakra energy recovery, it will help to envision the energy pristine, healthy and clear. You also wish to observe the energy swirling to you on a clockwise direction.

Take your time on this and also do not proceed to another Chakra until you feel that the present Chakra is healthy, energized and strong. As you proceed, don't block the flow of energy in the prior Chakra, let it keep energizing that Chakra. Following the crown Chakra till it is completed and imagine the energy out of all of the crystals recharging your Chakras until you feel it's complete.

Chakra energy recovery can be achieved together with the assistance of another individual if wanted. It's ideal to have someone you trust and feel a strong relationship with.

This is so that there's no negative energies introduced while doing the Chakra energy recovery. When you have finished the Chakra energy recovery, you need to ground yourself. Sit still for some moments and entangle once more to your environment.

Drink water and permit the Chakra power to stabilize. This Chakra energy recovery technique can be achieved daily if needed. As you practice this you will notice your own energy is increasing and you've got a fantastic general sense of health.

Chakra healing's artwork has been utilized for centuries to balance significant energy centers in our body known as Chakras. We can use quite a few unique tools such as meditation or stones throughout Chakra balancing. The final result will be a physically healthy body, a happier, more peaceful you.

Many people find out that bringing equilibrium in the kind of activities, self-reflections, meditation stability within the house, equilibrium inside one's life, and equilibrium with the daily diet and workout of one, will help you find good balance. Chakras cannot be bottled up, nevertheless our bodies soak them up and they greatly affect behaviors, emotions, feelings and our metabolism.

In addition to their purposes in the world, Chakras run on a higher plane, waking up into the understanding that our mind, body and soul are eternally and permanently linked. Whether you encounter pain, nervousness or illness, or only need to enhance your energy, you are going to know and exercise this simple-yet-profound technique.

Different dynamics might be employed to cure many diseases. You only say out what you would love to change - pain or the matter - and - tap, breathe deeply and feel how the body strain causing the distress melts off. The idea is that by touching 4 major points in your body when committing statements, you are surely in a place of stress induced disturbance in your body's healing energy.

It might sound easy, but the results tend to be profoundly transformative. Power moves in and out of Chakras which energize the body's bloodstream. Additionally, fueling the meridians, Chakras specifically supply the body cells, muscles, tissues, and organ systems with the power to flourish.

Since emotional and physical contaminants can block the Chakras, sometimes energy will become blocked or stagnant and the organ systems the Chakras feed become deficient. Maintaining the Chakras healthy and clean is essential in ensuring optimum physical health.

The 7 major Chakras not just fuel the actual physical body with electricity, they energize the mental body also. Each Chakra accounts for various emotions, thoughts, and perceptions correlating with elements of life. In reality, in many cases, it is the psychological part of our being that regulates the actual physical result.

What this means is that usually, it is an emotion or a psychological tie to a circumstance in life that leaves our Chakras depleted of power. Negative emotions are accountable for most of the poisonous clogs that result in the Chakras being partially blocked. Due to this particularity, several physical conditions or diseases are immediate results of many years of mental turmoil.

The challenging part with mental diseases is the absence of physical signs; which means they might not constantly be kept in the 1/6 of the human brain we use.

Instead, they're kept in the additional 5/6 of the brain, or the subconscious. The subconscious can store numerous past psychological disturbances that could not have registered consciously but have profoundly affected us on an energetic level.

The best part is you'll find ways to clean the unwanted subconscious beliefs calculated beliefs and the Chakra centers. There are many methods utilized by energy medicine practitioners to mend and restore balance to the

Chakras and also unravel damaging applications being kept in the mental faculties and body resulting in physical and emotional diseases.

CHAPTER 13

CHAKRAS, ENDOCRINE SYSTEM AND THE IMMUNE SYSTEM

The seven Chakras not just fuel the actual physical body with electricity, they energize the mental body also. Each Chakra accounts for various emotions, thoughts, and perceptions correlating with elements of life. In reality, in many cases, it is the psychological part of our being that regulates the actual physical end result.

What this means is that usually, it is an emotion or a psychological tie to a circumstance in life which leaves our Chakras depleted of power. Chakras, as stated previously, are actually energy hotspots all over the entire body which fuel the body's whole energetic method with divine energy (also known as chi or prana).

Given that everything in the world is made of matter and matter is made of power, science has proven that everything that surrounds us is actually made of energy. Chakras are the power centers present in all living things. Power moves in and out of Chakras, which energize the body's bloodstream.

Additionally, fueling the meridians, Chakras specifically supply the body cells, muscles, tissues, and organ systems with the power to flourish. Since emotional and physical contaminants can block the Chakras, sometimes energy will become blocked or stagnant and the organ systems the Chakras feed becomes deficient. Maintaining the Chakras healthy and clean is essential in ensuring optimum physical health.

Negative emotions are accountable for most of the poisonous clogs in the Chakras resulting in them being partially blocked. Due to this particularity, several physical conditions or diseases are an immediate result of many years of mental turmoil.

The subconscious can store numerous past psychological disturbances that could not have registered consciously but have profoundly affected you on an energetic level. The best part is you'll find ways to clean the unwanted subconscious beliefs and the Chakra centers.

There are amazing methods utilized by energy medicine practitioners to mend and restore balance to the Chakras and also unravel damaging applications being kept in the mental faculties and body resulting in physical and emotional diseases.

When you are in a state of health and vitality most of the 7 Chakras are connected, aligned, open, and flowing. In cases where they are closed, misaligned, stuck, or disconnected one could experience sickness of body, soul and mind. And so let us now get back to the six methods and five reasons Chakra healing can assist kids. Ways:

- Relaxing & Calming: A Chakra Healing Session is going to allow time for leisure and soothing. Time for a kid to chill out and relax a little can make an advantageous distinction for the health and wellbeing of the kid.

- Clarity & Increased Mental Focus: A Chakra Healing Session can market enhanced clarity and mental focus as the power starts to flow far more harmoniously and the brain is actually cleared and calmed. This clarity will even change into enhanced interaction for the kid.

- Clearing and releasing: A Chakra Healing Session supports a secure spot for releasing and clearing of emotions and toxins which are damaging for the kid, by being saved in the body tissues and energy field. As the Chakras align, balance, flow and clean it enables the whole being to be at peace.

- Self Awareness: During a Chakra Healing Session a kid is going to have a chance to talk about what they are experiencing and give feedback to ensure that they start making wholesome connections of exactly how certain patterns are actually impacting them.

- Positive Thought Patterns: Chakra Healing Sessions can support kids in purposely being conscious of how the thoughts are actually impacting their power flow and effort is carried out to help support the kid in selecting a lot more good feelings.

- Self Esteem: All of this goes in concert to allow a kid in having improved self-esteem and a far healthier, positive self-image and self-acceptance.

Reasons:

1. Balance: Balancing of the Chakras to allow a more harmonious flow of electricity will change the experience of the entire being: soul, mind and body.

2. Connection with Self: Chakra Healing enables the connection of all of the Chakras to one another, so they are operating as a good whole system

3. Connection with Source: This work additionally allows for integration and acknowledgment of the connection to a Source. The source is actually the divine energy which includes everything around and inside.

4. Grounding: Chakra Healing enables a crucial opportunity for the spiritual being to get healthily grounded in the physical vessel and the current moment of life.

5. Breathing: Chakra Healing also honors the gift of breath and also works for much more relaxed, present, useful breathing which will likely translate in a better general wellbeing.

Working with the Chakras during youth is a special chance to aid kids on the trip of life as they continue learning, develop, play, discover and find their place. It can really allow for the experience of youth to be healthy, connected and empowered.

Chakra Healing is a terrific chance to help kids in living and experiencing balanced, fulfilled and happier lives.

CHAPTER 14
OTHER METHODS TO HEAL THE CHAKRAS

Distant Energy Healing

This particular approach might seem uncommon to a lot of individuals though it's been used in the Far East for hundreds of years and today there are many contemporary techniques to do that.

More and more individuals are switching to alternative healing treatments such as distant Chakra healing to improve their wellbeing. Qigong healing is a potent method to help heal, align, clear, and balance the Chakras.

Qigong energy healing continues to be utilized effectively in the East and West to cure a bunch of psychological, emotional and physical problems and additionally extremely efficient in Chakra healing.

How does Qigong distant healing favorably impact the Chakras and other power routes from a distance? You will find locations including the California Pacific Medical Center and the Northern California Institute of Noetic

Sciences which have scientifically analyzed the usefulness of distant energy healing.

A rigid double-blind study with almost 400 individuals by cardiologist Robert Bryd, discovered that individuals who had been prayed for had better results compared to people who weren't. Quantum Physics might offer some answers to the reason why distant or remote healing works.

In the 1980's at the Faculty of Paris, some scientists led by Alain Aspect made an incredible discovery that could be the most essential one in contemporary science.

They discovered that under certain instances some subatomic particles had the ability to talk immediately with one another regardless of the distance they had been out of one another. It didn't matter in case they were large numbers of miles apart.

Nicolas Gisin duplicated the findings and concluded that several particles seemed to be talking at the amazing velocity of times 20,000 the pace of light. These conclusions might give clues as to how distance healing functions.

David Bohm, the quantum physicist surmises that the reason why subatomic particles can remain in connection with one another despite amazing distances isn't because they are transmitting a number of unfamiliar signals forth and back but because the splitting up of the debris is actually an illusion.

Bohm concludes that at a deeper level of truth the particles aren't specific entities but are extensions of the identical base and everything in the Universe is interconnected. Several scientists now tell what mystics from many countries have stated for a millennium that "we are many, not separate but profoundly interconnected".

Distance healing energy can be transferred through many distances since we are interconnected. It does not make any distinction when the one transmitting the power is in a distinct community or across the planet from the receiver. Distant Qigong energy healing is a really impressive way for Chakra healing and healing on the whole. It is been effective for many conditions.

It has been proven and tested to be helpful for pain and stress reduction, mental balancing, boosting stamina and immunity, and a large variety of some other health issues.

Magnet Therapy

Magnet Healing is starting to become one of the most popular means of healing, together with Chakra Therapy. You will find loads of advantages linked to these 2 therapies, which includes significantly greater oxygen flow and enhanced blood flow.

Speaking of such benefits, we can't help but note the Magnet Treatment and Rehabilitation. The advantages of Chakra Healing are of huge value, as it improves your wellness and wellbeing, psychologically, emotionally and physically. Chakras are in fact lightweight wheels that are situated all over the human body.

Right now, there are huge amounts of them almost everywhere in the body; however, the site of the seven major Chakras is actually on the backbone. The color of every Chakra is represented by a rainbow color - violet, yellow, green, blue, indigo, red and orange. These Chakras are believed to be psychic muscles and also places of hidden perspective, understanding and knowledge.

When there's Chakra imbalance, the condition impacts the complete wellbeing. Chakra Therapy discovers the imbalance explanation and also eliminates it. There are many solutions with regards to Chakra Therapy, but no matter the technique used, the healing can provide incredibly good outcomes.

How can the Magnet Treatment Help Me? Not so far in the past, the Magnet Healing was dismissed as a bad technique of healing, and what is even worse, it was seen as quackery. The skeptics believed that the advantages had been only a placebo effect.

Nevertheless, that's all changed right now, as you will find increasingly more scientific studies to prove that the Magnet Treatment is a good healing program. It is been proved it aided with several problems, including epilepsy, arthritis, spinal injuries, wound healing, depression, and incontinence, and furthermore, Magnet Treatment is being examined as a good treatment for lots of various other problems, including MS, cancer, and migraine.

The idea of utilizing magnets as therapeutic products isn't new. The Magnet Healing is perfectly advanced in

China, Japan, India, Australia and Germany, though various other countries as Holland, Canada, Great Britain and also the U.S. started to show interest in these healing methods.

The Concept behind the Magnet Rehabilitation Pain can impact everybody and, unfortunately, several individuals can't rely on medical treatment.

That is precisely why more individuals decide on natural healing techniques, including aroma massage therapy, and rehabilitation and hypnotherapy. Placing magnets on the injured area is quite advantageous since the magnetic field really assists the oxygen nutrients to encircle the injured region.

Here's a Chinese proverb that attractively links the lower Chakra triad with top of the Chakra triad through the heart Chakra: have a green bough at the center and the singing bird will appear.

This is a lovely reminder that in case you keep alive what is in the heart that's grounded in you, the song you hear will arrive in daily life. This is the secret that's encouraged by what is now familiar as the Law of Attraction.

This particular proverb starts with the guide to a green bough. The green bough is attached to the tree that gives life and this is how the power of life moves through you.

This is symbolic of being grounded in the human body and being free of emotional connections to family or tribal culture. This doesn't imply you abandon your connection to the family, clan or tribal culture; it does suggest you forgive the way you have been wounded by any attachment to them, that have limited you in expressing exactly who you are meant to be.

When you are grounded within the body and you have a connection to what the poet David Whyte refers to as living in a body in total presence, the bough will be greener, given that the origins of the tree aren't submerged in the bath of repressed emotions (second Chakra) or are actually burnt out by intensive emphasis of will to power (third Chakra). If the job of the lower Chakras is unfolded, the tree of life will develop green.

Green color is the sign of living and development. This particular greenness is actually the progress of the spirit. It is radically alive. This aliveness is the element attracting the experience of the singing bird. The singing bird is a metaphor for the soul. Without having immediate attention of the soul, you are as a tree growing in a desert.

You will have a strange sense of self and also the birds grouping the sky will be vultures. We come across this occurring in a world of competition. This is the motion from the will of power to the will to love. This is the crucial quest that's taking place on the planet nowadays.

Except if we, as people (and it starts with the individual) become well prepared to live through the will to really like the collective power can't be diverted from its over-focus on the will of power with the world of duality; this present society might as well ruin us as species. This is happening today. Most of us have had some experience type of singing bird.

Within fundamentalist religions the bird has its wings clipped and the positioned in a golden cage; the bird's song is currently recognized as a holy book. The singing bird is actually worshipped though it is not free to fly to the tree that gives life. In this particular cage of trust, the singing bird is only able to sing one specific note, which is hardly ever one of pleasure.

This is what the singer-songwriter Leonard Cohen implies as he creates The Holy dove, she'll be found once again. This holy dove represents the Holy Spirit.

This is an experience sensed throughout the heart. This is not about a cerebral belief. Just about all that one could then say is that one knows about the Holy Spirit, the holy dove or the singing bird.

The singing bird is actually perceived as a presence that turns into a body in total presence, an invitation to the experience of the transfiguration on Mount Sinai.

This is the experience of total embodiment. One really needs, in order to be grounded within the body, to invite Heaven on Earth and then to invite the will to Love to manifest.

Chakra Healing is basically a method of allowing. If you move out of the will of power to the will to Love you'll be lined up with the flow of allowing what is to be. You don't cage a singing bird inside a cage of words known as

Holy Scripture. The Holy Scripture becomes the way you are feeling the power move with the entire body.

The moment you would like to discover a few Holy Scriptures of presence, you may want to try that. But, unless you switch and become as kids, you won't ever type in the heavenly kingdom. - Matthew 18:3 Kids are actually the epitome of bodies in total presence.

Whenever we move out of the will of power to the will to Love the world's kids will be our most valuable resource since they are linked to the Source and remind us that's it exactly how we'll have all of the information about the life of the singing bird.

Solfeggio Frequencies, Modern Quantum physics are just now starting to know what the old wise males & mystics have told us for a huge number of years; that everything in the Universe such as ourselves, is actually in a continuous state of vibration. All have a peak range of maximum vibration and this range is actually widely known as being a resonance. Individual balance equals resonance.

Audio is an essential type of vibration, and you can make good use of this information to heal, you have to recognize that each cell and organ in the body emits and absorbs sound and has a specific resonance. an immediate and profound way to affect the resonance in body cells with sound is actually by utilizing the Chakras.

Mental states and emotions likewise have certain resonance frequencies; this is the transformational power behind religious music, mantras, and prayer. Mental states and emotions can also be attached to the Chakra audio wavelengths.

Whenever we expose a Chakra to its distinct noise frequency long enough, the Chakra is going to balance; and when these Chakras are in balance, same happens to the body mind and soul. Solfeggio frequencies are the initial sound frequencies utilized in Gregorian Chants.

The Gregorian chants and the distinct Solfeggio wavelengths are found to convey deep religious blessings when sung in balance and harmony. The Solfeggio wavelengths are thought to possess numerous psycho-spiritual and physical healing attributes. For a good example, 528Hz correlates to the note "MI" in the contemporary Western musical scale.

The frequencies also match with the healing Chakra sounds, with the Crown Chakra thus resonating at 960Hz. I use the Chakra affiliated Solfeggio frequencies, together with Tibetan singing bowls, to heal soul, mind, and body. The Tibetan singing bowls are utilized for deep breathing.

A number of people think these were utilized entirely for meditation, while others think these were resources for the sensational transformation of self and of matter.

The organic and natural sound is unparalleled for evoking a trance state, and by utilizing Tibetan singing bowls attuned to the Chakras, we can evoke a full transformation of the entire body, soul and mind.

CHAPTER 15

HEALING POWER OF REIKI

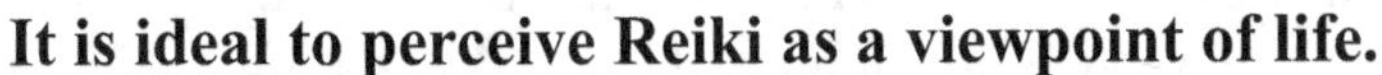

It is ideal to perceive Reiki as a viewpoint of life.

There's no mystery to Reiki, especially Western Reiki. With standard Reiki, there's a bit more secrecy, with intuition driving the positioning of the hands in a Reiki healing session, for instance. Defined hand placements are utilized at the Western type of Reiki.

Due to that, it is less difficult to study and understand the healing techniques of the Western type. A therapy is no higher than a session to make an attempt to attain energy stability to enhance the flow of life force with the entire body. Reiki and quantum physics share the idea of exactly how energy flows and interacts.

If appropriate alignment and balancing are actually attained for the big energy routes of the entire body, then the flow of the common life force is actually enhanced.

Several healers make use of the ideal mixture of sounds and symbols. Chakra healing prescribes particular gemstones & crystals and also specific styles, to help with balancing a certain Chakra.

Emotional and physical attributes are affected or managed by each Chakra. Usui, the founding father of Reiki, didn't particularly relate to these Chakras in his Reiki application, though we are aware he integrated a lot of the old healing techniques that deal with the way energy moves through the entire body. Self-application of Reiki therapies is achievable.

It can additionally be used to mend and balance others. As a pupil advances by instruction, the ability to remotely heal is taught and learned Throughout a Reiki healing session, the master might endeavor to balance all of the Chakras. She or he might also concentrate on one or 2, based on the reason behind the treatment.

Based on the disorder or illness, just several of the Chakras might seem to the professional to be out of balance. Seeing a Reiki treatment is certainly eye-opening. Lots of skeptical opinions have been swayed by the crystal-clear enhancement of the affected person and the aura of serenity and wellbeing after a consultation. By getting attuned to Reiki and studying, you can dispose the blocks into the Chakra in a way.

In some cases, receiving the attunements of reiki only will rid of the blocks out of the Chakra opening the channel. Love, intelligence and light are the basis of energy. Your thoughts are in control of the energy flow inside you. Different energy centers inside your body are affected by your thoughts and habits. In other words - money, spirituality, your energy centers - impact.

These energy centers known as your Chakras and these Chakras may balance via Reiki Self Attunement. Below are free exercises to help balance your mind through Reiki.

1. The White Light: In the eye of your mind, see a crystal - white light. Make this light as bright as you can imagine.

See and feel the light passing through the inside of the top of your head, clearing any negative and dark thoughts from the crown Chakra. Allow the traveling through your body and envision all darkness being cleared out throughout all the Chakras. Once you concluded the meditation, you should imagine your Chakras perfectly balanced and illuminated in proportion.

2. Breathing Colors: Picture yourself breathing in green, as you focus on a a deep breath. Find yourself inhaling yellow as you exhale. Breathe in blue as deep as you can and breathe out orange. Draw in purple visualizing the purple penetrating every cell of your blood. Finally, breathe red completely out.

Repeat this meditation process three times.

3. Glass Globes: Picture eight glass globes piled together with one another. The globes are stacked from the top to base; Royal-Purple, Red-Violet, Deep Blue, Emerald Green, Sunshine Yellow, Sky Blue, Vivid Orange and Ruby Red. See the globes become larger, brighter and illuminated. Make them expand in size till they are large.

See the globes totally translucent and colors as apparent, with no spots present on the glass.

These 3 exercises are perfect for beginners that are hoping to balance their Chakras. This self-attunement with reiki will help one heal every time of the day, balance and clear Chakras and learn meditation.

As you get more energy sensitivity, you can start a complex healing pattern. Determine which Chakras need to be energized by scanning with a pendulum.

The procedure can be performed by putting one hand on a weak Chakra and the other on the Chakra on top of it for 3 minutes. This derives energy from a stronger Chakra to elevate the power of the weaker one. Proceed to connect the feeble Chakra to all the Chakras below.

To summarize the procedure, review this example for connecting the heart Chakra to the top Chakras: left hand on center, right hand over the throat; left hand on center, right hand on the forehead; left hand on center, right hand on the crown.

Now, join the heart Chakra with the lower Chakras: right hand on the heart, left hand plexus; right hand on the heart, left hand on the throat Chakra; right hand on center, left hand above the root Chakra. This completes the relationship of the heart with the other Chakras, thus absorbing energy from them all.

When connecting the Chakras, consider the following implications. For instance, when connecting the heart Chakra to the other Chakras, some questions could direct your therapeutic communicating: What would you like to express on your emotions?

How can you feel about your creative expression? What do you believe (Chakra 4) about your actions (Chakra 3)? What action can you take (Chakra 3) to handle your emotions (Chakra 4)? Connecting the Chakras could be a very potent way to round out your personality.

After reviewing the features of all the Chakras, you'll get a better idea of your strengths and flaws. If you discover that the solar plexus is highly charged as signified by very large self-confidence plus a highly driven character, this implies an excess of energy in your next Chakra. If you discover that you have tumors or cysts in the reproductive system, this indicates a closed or weak second Chakra.

By assessing your physical symptoms and personal traits, you determine which Chakras need connection and healing.

Chakra Spread –

This technique can be used for acute emotional or body pain. It brings a person to a deeper level of recovery than most other techniques. It should be reserved for special needs and sacred moments in healing. Make sure your patient sits in a chair while you're standing in front of them.

Start by grounding yourself well - emotionally stable and physically anchored to the ground. Put your palms on your patient's feet for some minutes to make sure they stood firm on the ground. Then hold their hands in your own for up to two minutes to start their hands Chakras. Walk behind them and place both palms on their crown.

Open their crown Chakra by softly and gradually lifting both of your palms out and up as far as you can reach, such as the wings of an eagle. Perform this motion three times. If other folks have need of opening, disperse them in precisely the exact same method. Reiki healing basically consists of hands-on solutions created to enhance the flow of good energy with the entire body.

Chakras channel the energy moves and appropriated Chakra healing is integrated by numerous healers. Bad weather of (rei) life force (ki) is exactly where the term Reiki comes from. It makes good sense that the energy around us and flowing through us has healing attributes.

Ailments and illness can happen with poor or sub-optimal power flow. In the entire therapy, the Reiki practitioner is going to ask the individual to stretch on the massage table. Loose and comfortable clothes are used by the patient. Before the process, the professional is going to meditate to be mentally ready for the treatment.

The practitioner might also make use of the non-touching method, exactly where the hands are kept very few centimeters from the body. The hands and wrists remain on each component of the body for 3 to 5 minutes before proceeding to various parts of the entire body. Reiki therapy could be practiced at a distance.

The Reiki master can do the distance healing by focusing on the spot they wish to deal with and delivering the power to it. Presently the alternative healing techniques are popular and one of the very popular types of alternative healing is the Reiki Chakra.

How is Reiki Chakra used to fix the power of the entire body? As stated before, you will find 7 main Chakras within the body and Reiki master use them to deal with nearly every ailment of the entire body.

Because the Chakras are positioned from head to toes and from the front to the back, the Reiki master starts the therapy at the crown Chakra. Several practitioners state that Reiki therapy uses Chakras to get common power. As of today, of all the alternative healing techniques the Reiki Chakra technique is discovered to be the best.

The Reiki Chakra technique is regarded as the well-known alternative healing method in the western nations. The crown Chakra is the divine Chakra, connecting one to sacred peace and universal energy. It is also not surprising that in several Asian cultures, it is inappropriate to touch the roof of the head, particularly on an older man or woman.

Have this in mind that when offering healing. It may be better to cradle the head from behind, instead of exclusively touching the crown, to have respect for an individual's divine center. The identity of this Chakra is common. Meditation is designed to transcend the little private ego of deference to a common self.

Operating out of this amount of being, the orientation reaches wisdom and transcendence. "Self" takes on an extremely different meaning than it did when we were kids and the solar plexus was just starting to blossom. The crown Chakra tunes us into a "universal self." Typical ailments related to the crown Chakra include coma, amnesia, and migraines.

Deficiency in the crown Chakra could indicate extraordinary power of the lower Chakras manifesting as greed or materialism.

Location: Cerebral cortex, upper part of the skull.

Healing Color: Violet.

Element: Wisdom.

Age of Development: Early adulthood.

Individual Rights: To know and to learn.

Associated Physical Organs: Brain, the pineal gland.

Balanced Characteristics: Analytical, smart, innovative, open-minded, wise.

Signs of Deficiency: Spiritual cynicism, rigid beliefs, materialism.

Signs of Excess: Intellectualization, religious addiction, confusion.

Psychological Traumas: Forced religiosity, insured obedience.

Healing Practices: Meditation, examine belief system.

Positive Affirmation: I'm guided by my inner wisdom.

Another perspective concerning spiritual growth is explained extremely well by Chogyam Trungpa. He says, "the ego has the capacity to turn everything to personal use, even spirituality".

We must step out of ego's constant desire for a greater, much more religious, much more transcendental wy of expertise, religion or whatever the ego is seeking. The impulse of trying to find food is actually a hang-up. These words of warning are handy in case you fall into the trap of religious addiction.

I, undoubtedly, am a perfectionist. And so, I must pay heed to this particular problem, being very careful not to push Reiki and stay away from criticizing individuals that do not trust it. My private growth additionally demands I do not push myself way too much to be spiritual while keeping my ego in check moment by moment.

You have most likely met folks that do not have confidence in any religion, meditation or healing energy. Religious cynicism isn't always bad; it simply shows a deficiency of power at the crown Chakra

This is a great illustration of when we should be cautious not to push Reiki on anyone. We have to respect individuals as they are and for whatever they think.

There is lots of points in looking to persuade an individual to have confidence in Experience or Reiki since they just aren't at that moment in lives where such issues are essential to them. It will be like persuading a teenager that enjoys rap music to listen to one of Verdi's operas.

Let folks believe whatever they think and love what they love. In case the topic does develop in discussion with an individual with strong doubts about Reiki, it can be a good idea to describe it in phrases of quantum physics, instead of in terms of Chakras, to help keep the discussion much more concrete and technical instead of mystical.

Moreover, bear in your mind that you are under no obligation to explain Reiki to anyone. Just saying, "It is like meditating" could be adequate to lightly bring closure to the subject when needed. You can provide Reiki in the meditation practice and relaxation in the Reiki practice by focusing the efforts on the crown Chakra.

Connecting Your Chakras Using Reiki as you get sensitized to energy, you will start a more complex healing pattern. Determine the Chakra's need to be energized by using a pendulum. The procedure can be performed by putting a hand on a weak Chakra and the other on the Chakra on top of it for 3 minutes.

This derives energy from a stronger Chakra to elevate the power of the weaker one. Keep your hands on that weak Chakra when moving another hand on one more Chakra until the energy stabilizes. Do this for every Chakra above, all the way to the crown. Proceed to connect the feeble Chakra to all the Chakras below.

Keep one hand on the weak Chakra and put your other hand on each of the Chakras below until all the Chakras are attached to the weak one. To summarize the procedure, review this example for connecting the heart Chakra to the top Chakras.

After reviewing the features of all the Chakras, you'll get a better idea of your strengths and flaws. If you discover that your solar plexus is highly charged as signified by considerable self-confidence plus a highly driven character, this implies an excess of energy in your next Chakra. At the same time, if you discover that you have cysts or tumors on your reproductive system, this indicates a weak or closed second Chakra.

By assessing your personal traits and physical symptoms, determine which Chakras are in need of healing and connection.

CHAPTER 16
HEALING POWER OF CRYSTALS

Crystals are universal energies that allow you to get the individual energies into integration and healing.

Each crystal comprises their own "character" and can also be utilized in unique techniques to assist comprehension of nature presence on Earth. Crystals are nature's gift to mankind and can be found in all sizes, shapes, colors and composition.

They each have a distinctive vibrational resonance due to their varying mineral materials, their inherent geometry and the color frequency they exude; hence they may be powerful recovery tools.

Crystal healing is a method whereby gemstones are put on the body, utilized as reflex tools to stimulate points on the feet, worn, or could be placed around one's home to boost Feng Shui energy.

They heal on physical, mental, emotional and spiritual levels, helping to guide the flow of energy to a particular portion of the body, restore balance and finally cleanse by releasing blocked energy.

The vibration of body energy is an electromagnetic system which the crystals are also capable of interacting with because they're nature's best electromagnetic conductors. Crystals work through resonance and have been discovered to carry vibrations that trigger specific energy centers, favorably affecting our body system.

Some crystals also contain minerals known for their curative abilities used in medical practices. They're piezoelectric, meaning light and power is produced by compression and can produce sound waves. Choosing a crystal to utilize can be as straightforward as following your instinct about what captures the gist of energy you're drawn to, or you can reference crystal recovery indicators to help you associate symptoms with relevant crystals.

These beings that are powerful are sacred tools to encourage us on our individual journeys and serve as route to harmonious balance, higher consciousness, personal evolution, well-being, subconscious unveiling and healing support. Crystal healing is celestial clarity that must be activated by an alchemical process that blends crystal energy with our core vibration.

Individuals have always been drawn to Crystals, primarily because of their visual appeal, exquisite purity, fantastic interplay of colors and also "crystal-clear" transparency. Crystals and precious stones have outstanding features, making them convenient to be used as tools in different metaphysical, spiritual and therapeutic practices.

The spiritual science believes that living beings which are at the simple level of development of consciousness and crystals are all members of the mineral kingdom. This is compared to the belief that is widely spread based on todays' science parameters in which crystals are not categorized as living entities. Various vibration crystals are also capable of collecting energy.

Furthermore, they can boost the energy and bring it back to our environment through vibration and resonance. After we've mastered the communication art with our crystals, they are going to reveal to us more - their hidden virtues and qualities.

It's believed that the religious basis of coping with crystals originates from Atlantis, where a potent technology for obtaining crystals synthetically has been invented, allowing production of crystals in extended proportions for different purposes. Amidst the number of crystals that are available, it might be hard for us to choose the ideal crystal.

There are many essential points in picking crystals which should be considered before creating our thoughts, for example visual appeal, intuitive appeal and attraction at crystal's practical values. Once the crystal has been chosen, for instance by using the help of one of the 4 elements (fire, water, earth and air) we can start learning to control and use it.

By charging, we associate it with all the types and qualities of energy we would like to place within our crystal.

By programming, we augment our selected intentions, feelings, and thoughts to the crystal energy routine and our crystal will enhance and irradiate them back to us. The color of crystals can be a fantastic indication as to what sort of metaphysical clinic or therapeutic practice their specific energies are acceptable for.

For example, white or purple crystals open the doorway of perception, bring unity. Red crystals are symbols of life, vitality, power. Energies are moved by them, they worm up.

Life is encouraged by orange crystals energy, that support self-control and regulate the performance of the glands. Yellow crystals influence the functioning of the gallbladder, kidneys, the liver and spleen and also assist digestion.

Green crystals represent the color of harmony, health, and love. They help to regulate our blood pressure, heart disorders, stimulate love and calm the nerves. Ultimately, it's important to remember that crystals occupy the omnipresent cosmic love, spreading their continuous vibrations of energy and amplifying it.

They've been supporting God's production, by outpouring their spirituality and love to the world, transmitting the Sun's light, love and warmth and, along with it, their structural stability. Because of this, it is comforting to know they can be our devoted friends, teachers and advisers.

Crystals as An Alchemy for the Soul

The Earth consciousness supports humanity's awakening to re-discovery of ancient healing arts, such as crystals.

Think of the Chakras as a backyard, with each flower needing care. While others are more demanding, some will require less care. The self-scrutiny dedication makes Chakras healing challenging as it's rewarding. The guidelines below can be altered to your needs. When picking stones, be attentive not to the size or appearance, but rather to your reaction.

Some of these crystals may not feel familiar, but you are likely to see them at a metaphysical store. Although you may enjoy this introduction to Chakra healing, it is ideal to undertake treatment with the advice of a trained practitioner. Besides having the experience, many expert website healers are intuitive. Their insight might help you to understand the reasons.

1st Chakra:

This is the main Chakra. It is found at the lower part of the tailbone or spine. The root Chakra also belongs to the physical realm. This spectacle requires attention if you feel protected, grounded and rooted in the present. Many aren't so blessed. A root Chakra that is blocked may direct one to grasp in the physical, becoming clingy and possessive.

Conversely, if you open here you will feel estranged from possessions and your body. As a result, people may be taking advantage of your generosity.

Crystal Correction: A blocked root Chakra can be opened by using obsidian. So, the impulse acquired is substituted by understanding the nature of possessions. This gem brings a focused, peaceful perspective.

To heal blocks, place an obsidian on your genital area whilst lying down on your back, as you unwind more the strength of the stone and your own will connects, enhancing it.

Quartz rose

This pink quartz permits us to love ourselves, so we can protect ourselves though typically linked to the heart.

Sacral Chakra

The sacral Chakra regulates creativity and our power. You need to press at just two inches below your navel. A balanced Chakra means dash and expressiveness.

A blockage may lead to resistance to unique ideas. A sacral Chakra that is very open is evident and it manifests as reckless behavior, from dangerous driving to bed-hopping.

The Crystal Correction: Carnelian - this beautiful quartz is for opening the sacral center.

The stimulating qualities of orange or red give us courage. This allows us to pursue our great dreams, without any fear-based illusions obstructing our path.

Conversely, if the Chakra really is too open, we might want to use luizi crystals. This blue stone was valued in Babylon and ancient Egypt. We can utilize its properties to help us act with caution.

Only touching your system with this rock improves your spiritual, psychic, mental, physical and psychological condition. For optimal benefits to the Chakra, rest this stone as desired.

Solar Plexus Chakra

This Chakra is also known as the energy center. This resides a reservoir of heroism and untapped will. When this solar plexus Chakra is wholesome, our potential is really motivated to explore.

When it is blocked, we feel as if we have "butterflies in our stomach" or experience additional stomach woes. An energy center that is obstructed makes us behave and feel helpless. When this energy-center is too broad, the opposite problem happens.

Crystal Correction: Golden Beryl is a mild, orange yellow stone which directs will and boosts confidence. It is excellent for Chakra blockages.

Placing this rock 2 inches above the navel will free your power center. For people overwhelmed by this Chakra jade is adequate. This calming stone reduces impulses towards other people and helps stock our fires gently.

Heart Chakra

This really is the heart Chakra and it is self-explanatory. It is the celestial world of spiritual growth, high ideals, love and resilience.

A heart Chakra that is congested makes us critical of both ourselves and others. In this condition, we find it difficult to open ourselves to possibilities for friendships and love. Contrarily, if our heart is too big, we might attempt to do the impossible, trying to take the weight of the Earth.

Crystal Correction: The green jasper helps us feel secure to open up and show ourselves. This eases joyful and honest communication. To get a heart with no bounds, it's advisable you try using peridots. This pastel rock recharges us. Peridot allows us to be unsacrificial and sympathetic.

Throat Chakra

This Chakra aids in communicating in both spoken and body language. It's situated at the lower part of the throat.

When this Chakra is balanced, we talk honestly.

Correction: Sodalite crystal is a stunning navy rock that helps to ease a throat that is constricted. This crystal promises clarity and courage.

On the other hand, people who have a 5th Chakra have to speak the truth quietly. Amber can be helpful within this capacity.

Brow Center Chakra – You Most know this energy center between the brows as "the third eye".

If in equilibrium, this Chakra gives us the capability to show our innate psychic capacity. But we limit ourselves to unproven facts when it is obstructed. This also leads to thinking that is stiff and disrupted. If we're too open here we may be disconnected from the physical world.

Correction: A moonstone located on the brow center Chakra clears the issues that blindfolded our intuition and directly opens our mind thus embracing personal development, because moonstone is connected to cycles of change.

This helps us tune in to stream, welcoming spontaneity and discharging rigidity. With an open eye, blue agate is required. This sky-blue crystal stone clears out the mess of distraction and sharpens our attention.

Crown Center Chakra

Words aren't enough to express the profound capacity of the crown Chakra. This Chakra represents enlightenment. Even though balancing the Chakra can't make us a Buddha, it will certainly take us to peaks of bliss and connect with the purpose of our life. You are far from alone, if you are blocked here.

We might be confused about our career when blocked and lack calmness that was, rapturous, that was lasting. For maximum results at balancing this Chakra, we must ensure the wellbeing of our prior Chakras. If you don't dislike stability and joy, possessing this Chakra is an issue.

We can communicate with the sorrowful and cynic. Otherwise we are trapped in our own mind which could get lonely. The clear quartz is a perfect healer for a lot of Chakras and particularly useful for opening a closed crown. Due to the Chakra's place, the crystal chosen should be modest enough to rest on your head.

This stone offers clarity of purpose and makes it possible for us to see the meaning. It guides us to comprehend and live with truths. For all those with an open crown Chakra, hematite is perfect. By drawing attention, this stone helps us fulfill our own earthly needs.

CONCLUSION

As a beginner, you can think of each Chakra as various areas of yourself: from bottom to top: 1st - your base; 2nd - your physical needs and desires; 3rd - your self-esteem and empowerment; 4th - your feelings and emotions; 5th - your need to vocalize your dreams and convey your beliefs; 6th - your intuition and instincts; 7th - your soul and connection to our world and Higher Awareness.

Chakras, as stated previously, are energy hotspots all over the body, which fuel the body with divine energy (also known as chi or prana). Given that everything on the world is made of matter, and matter is made of power, we can conclude that everything on Earth is energy. Chakras are the power centers present in all living things.

Power moves in and out of Chakras which energizes the body, fueling the meridians. Chakras specifically supply the body cells, muscles, tissues and organ systems with the power to flourish.

Maintaining the Chakras healthy and clean is essential in ensuring optimum physical health. The seven major Chakras not just fuel the actual physical body with energy, they also energize the mental body.

Each Chakra accounts for various emotions, thoughts and perceptions correlating with elements of life. All in all, in many cases, it is the psychological part of our being that regulates the actual physical end result. What this means is that usually, it is an emotion or a psychological tie to a circumstance in life that leaves our Chakras depleted of power.

Negative emotions are accountable for most of the poisonous clogs that come in the Chakras being partially blocked. Due to this particularity, several physical conditions or body diseases are an immediate result of many years of mental turmoil. The challenging part with psychological diseases is the lack of physical pain; which means that it is our subconscious brain that keeps track of them.

The subconscious can store numerous past psychological disturbances that could not have registered consciously but have profoundly affected us on an energetic level. The best part is you'll find ways to clean the unwanted subconscious beliefs and the Chakra centers.

There are methods utilized by energy medicine practitioners to mend and restore balance to the Chakras and unravel damaging applications being kept in the mental faculties and body resulting in physical and emotional disease. This specific strategy is ideal for maintaining your Chakras balanced & clear.

It is proven that crystals have a comparable crystalline framework as the body. Consequently, in case you set minerals and gemstones in proximity, your body can easily absorb the healing vibrations. Furthermore, it is an undeniable fact that all of the Chakras resonate at frequencies that are various as do crystals.

This implies you can enjoy the advantages of picking the appropriate crystal for each Chakra and achieving maximum harmony inside of your system. What makes an unhealthy person ill is a faulty Chakra. At every node, Chakras have a certain frequency and if this frequency is disturbed, you develop a disease in that area.

Taking good care of your Chakra system will help to optimize your energy flow so that you can make the most out of your days.